more . . .

"No one ever found a thyroid problem. Thank goodness Dr. Siegal realized what the problem was. I've lost 65 pounds. I don't even recognize myself when I look in the mirror. I can't believe it!"

— Myra Garcia

"I went to Dr. Siegal last July because of his reputation for getting weight off his patients. I never dreamed that my other problems might be helped. I started taking thyroid hormones in August and I no longer have those horrendous mood swings. I sleep better, and best of all, I'm losing weight steadily."

— Cindy Kirsh

• • •

WHAT READERS ARE SAYING ABOUT
IS YOUR THYROID MAKING YOU FAT?

"If after you've read this book, taken all the tests, filled out the checklists, kept track of your temperature, and tried his 28-day eating test, you don't think you got your money's worth I'd be surprised....Dr. Siegal also gives strong arguments for the use of natural thyroid supplementation as opposed to the use of synthetics."

— Amy Shellase

"This book is great—I am giving it to my daughters to read, as they have a similar problem as me and are getting fed up with doctors who only go by lab results. Thanks for giving me some hope and having the courage to speak out against the 'establishment.' Wish there were more like Dr. Siegal."

— Roslyn Hodgins, Hammondville, NSW, Australia

"As a doctor of pharmacy candidate and published reviewer of medical literature, I am in constant contact with patients who complain that their doctor dismisses a metabolic problem as the cause of their obesity. While hypothyroidism certainly is not the cause of all obesity, Dr. Siegal makes a very convincing argument that, for many, it may be....This book offers hope to those who don't overeat but can't seem to lose weight on any diet."

— S. Hileman, Ft. Lauderdale, FL

IS YOUR THYROID MAKING YOU FAT?

The Doctor's 28-Day Diet that Tests Your Metabolism as You Lose Weight

---

Sanford Siegal, D.O., M.D.

WARNER BOOKS

A Time Warner Company

The information herein is not intended to replace the medical advice of your physician. You are advised to consult your health-care professional with regard to matters relating to your health, and in particular regarding matters that may require diagnosis or medical attention.

Copyright © 2000 by Sanford Siegal
All rights reserved.
No part of this book may be reproduced in any form or by any electronic or mechanical means, including information storage and retrieval systems, without permission in writing from the publisher, except by a reviewer who may quote brief passages in a review.

Warner Books, Inc., 1271 Avenue of the Americas,
New York, NY 10020

Visit our Web site at www.twbookmark.com

A Time Warner Company

Printed in the United States of America

Originally published in hardcover by Warner Books, Inc.
First Trade Printing: March 2001

10 9 8 7 6 5 4 3 2

The Library of Congress has cataloged the hardcover edition as follows:
Siegal, Sanford.
    Is your thyroid making you fat: the doctor's 28-day diet that tests your metabolism as you lose weight / Sanford Siegal
        p. cm.
    Includes bibliographical references and index.
    ISBN 0-446-52659-2
    1. Weight loss. 2. Hypothyroidism—Diagnosis. 3. Basal metabolism. 4. Thyroid gland function tests. I. Title.

RM222.2 .S533 2000
616.4'4—dc21

99-057900

ISBN 0-446-67710-8

Cover design by Mike Stomberg

Acknowledgments

Many people helped write this book; in a sense, thousands. They are the patients I've known for the last forty years.

Of the more recent contributors, I sincerely thank: my wife, Lyndol, for keeping my enthusiasm manageable; my friend, Peter Nguyen, for allowing me access to his knowledge of the biological world; my friends, Carmen and Greg Anderson, for their sage advice; my editor, Rick Horgan, for keeping me focused; my agent, Barbara Lowenstein, for her encouragement; my copy editor, Karen Thompson, for possessing the eye of an eagle; my son Marc Siegal, for making incomprehensible databases comprehensible; another son, Matthew Siegal, for his treasure chest of suggestions; a third son, Jason Siegal, for his critical input; and two great people, Cindy Hernandez and Beth Geisler, for dedicated slavery.

Contents

Appendices

Foreword

by Alan R. Gaby, M.D.

In this book, Dr. Sanford Siegal argues that hypothyroidism (underactive thyroid) is a common condition that is frequently overlooked by the average doctor. While conventional medicine relies primarily on blood tests to diagnose hypothyroidism, Dr. Siegal points out that these tests are unreliable and often fail to detect the problem. Siegal further differs from most doctors by recommending the use of desiccated thyroid, an extract from animal thyroid glands that modern medicine has repeatedly labeled "obsolete."

While most doctors are strongly opposed to—or even horrified by—the idea of giving a potent hormone to people whose blood tests are normal, my own clinical experience with more than a thousand "thyroid cases" unequivocally confirms Dr. Siegal's observations. Moreover, while only about 30 percent of patients can tell the difference between desiccated thyroid and the most frequently prescribed form of thyroid hormone (levothyroxine), those who *can* tell the difference nearly always prefer the natural preparation.

The symptoms of hypothyroidism are well known and include

fatigue, depression, constipation, cold hands and feet, dry skin, fluid retention, slow thinking, weight gain, menstrual irregularities, and an increase in serum cholesterol. Although these symptoms can have many different causes, I've found hypothyroidism to be one of the most common causes. And yet, approximately 85 percent of my patients whose symptoms improved (often dramatically) with thyroid treatment had normal thyroid blood tests, including TSH (thyroid-stimulating hormone).

The idea that blood tests often fail to detect hypothyroidism is not as far-fetched as it might seem. By analogy, many diabetics require injections of insulin, even though the level of this hormone in the bloodstream may be normal or above normal. This phenomenon is known as insulin resistance. While there is plenty of insulin circulating in the blood, the hormone receptors on cell membranes are inefficient in responding to insulin's message. As a result, some diabetics require higher-than-normal concentrations of insulin in their bloodstream in order to achieve a normal insulin effect. Thyroid-hormone resistance is also known to occur, although it is thought to be a rare condition. However, it is possible that a more subtle form of thyroid-hormone resistance is present in a relatively large proportion of the population. If that is the case, then some individuals would need to maintain their thyroid hormone level near the top of the normal range in order to feel well. While the existence of subtle thyroid-hormone resistance has not been proven, it could explain the dramatic results seen by Dr. Siegal, myself, and hundreds of other doctors who diagnose and treat hypothyroidism on clinical grounds.

Nor should it be surprising that desiccated thyroid works better for some individuals than does synthetic levothyroxine. The former contains two different molecules with known hormonal effects and two other compounds whose functions are unknown, whereas the latter contains only one of these four molecules.

Doctors who oppose the use of thyroid hormone on clinical grounds and rely instead on blood tests point out that inappropriate use of thyroid hormones can put stress on the heart and promote the development of osteoporosis (bone loss). While it's true that overtreatment can cause these problems, I would argue that empirical use of thyroid extract, when done carefully, is neither inappropriate nor overtreatment. I have not seen any cardiac problems with thyroid therapy, although a few patients developed chest pain, which was resolved when the dosage was reduced. Nor have my patients shown any evidence of accelerated osteoporosis, although, to be on the safe side, I always recommend a bone-building nutritional supplement along with thyroid hormone.

Dr. Siegal deserves to be commended for prescribing thyroid hormone the way he does and for having the courage to write about it.

Alan R. Gaby, M.D.
Past President of the American Holistic Medical Association
and author of *The Patient's Book of Natural Healing* and
Preventing and Reversing Osteoporosis
Seattle, Washington
November 1999

Foreword

by Stephen E. Langer, M.D.

World-famous actor-director Woody Allen once said, "The brain is my second favorite organ." If, as I suspect, his *favorite* organ is the thyroid gland, we agree.

The thyroid is a butterfly-shaped organ in the neck that releases approximately one ounce of hormone a year. This hormone controls the metabolism of every cell in the body, from your hair follicles to your toenails, and is as necessary for life as food and oxygen. I learned decades ago from my mentor, Dr. Broda Barnes (whom I consider the father of modern thyroid medicine), that as many as 40 percent of the American public are suffering from undetected hypothyroidism (underactive thyroid), and that relying on thyroid blood tests (T3, T4, FTI, TSH) for a diagnosis is misleading and often unsuccessful.

In the book you're about to read, Dr. Siegal discusses Dr. Barnes's Basal Temperature Test (which Dr. Barnes published in a *JAMA* article and which was promptly forgotten) and shares his own metabolic function index (MFI), which can be performed by anyone—at home, and without cost. This test can frequently serve as a much more sensitive indication of an underactive thyroid than the most commonly used laboratory tests.

A good doctor, however, should look at *all* the evidence: i.e., he or she should perform a thorough medical history and physical examination, and do all appropriate lab work—including the

Barnes test and the MFI—and only then rely on his or her own best clinical judgment as to whether or not supplemental thyroid is appropriate (usually it is).

In all my years of practicing preventive medicine, clinical nutrition, and anti-aging, I have found that prescribing thyroid medication when appropriate to patients suffering from the chronic problems enumerated in this book is the most important thing I can do to help my patients get well.

Without thyroid treatment, eating the best food and taking handfuls of nutritional supplements are wasted. Because of a sluggish metabolism, digestion suffers and the immune system does not perform optimally. A typical hypothyroid patient is therefore exhausted, prone to infections, overweight, has poor concentration, and suffers with many of the dozens of other symptoms known to accompany an underactive thyroid gland. The chronic debilitating symptoms of hypothyroidism are often misdiagnosed as chronic depression and treated with powerful antidepressant medication rather than thyroid hormone. This is not only wrong, it trivializes and patronizes a sick patient.

When a patient is placed on a small dose of thyroid hormone and gets appropriate medication and nutritional counseling, chronic problems like recurrent infections, migraine headaches, fibromyalgia, joint pain, high cholesterol, menstrual irregularities, acne and eczema, depression, and many others disappear like ice in the hot sun.

If it seems like I'm rhapsodizing about the benefits of supplemental "natural" thyroid, I am—it's often the Rosetta Stone of good health and should not be overlooked or underestimated. *Is Your Thyroid Making You Fat?* makes a valuable contribution to the thyroid literature.

Stephen E. Langer, M.D.
President of the American Nutritional Medical Association
and author of *Solved: The Riddle of Illness*
Berkeley, California
November 1999

Author's Note

In this age of political correctness, to avoid the appearance of gender bias, I might very well have written something like this:

> "I always instruct a new patient that when he or she consults his or her family doctor, he or she must inform him or her of exactly what medications I have prescribed for him or her."

That's probably more pronouns than you can tolerate at one sitting, hence I've decided to adopt the following approach: Since most of my patients are female, I've referred to the generic patient as *she*. However, since male physicians still outnumber females, doctors are referred to as *he*.

All of the tales of my patients are true, though to protect their privacy, I have used only first names and they are all pseudonyms. Where both a first and a last name are used, the name is real.

Dr. I. M. Conformist in Chapter 16 exists only in my imagination.

Preface

I'm a practical man.

That's not to say that I don't sometimes do silly things, that I don't indulge in fantasies, that I don't take chances. But more often than not, I'm practical. I try to do what reason tells me is the best choice, the thing that is most apt to succeed. That aspect of my personality probably operates even more rigidly in my medical practice than in my personal life. This makes sense to me. I'm dealing with the well-being of my patients, and that is an area where I shouldn't let my emotions get in the way of my good sense.

I try to do for them what works. This book is about what works. Specifically, it is about the method I've developed for evaluating and treating people who are overweight, with the goal of improving their health. I've long since accepted that I can best do this by helping them to achieve a normal weight and to do it safely. I believe that my methods are practical.

We're bombarded with weight-loss diets. They come from every source imaginable: books, magazine articles, the Internet, the government, commercial "clinics," and, yes, even doctors. Many are based on theories. Sometimes these theories are stated in terms designed to make us believe they are facts. Researchers publish scads of scientific papers that are intended to add to the total knowledge of the subject, and doctors pick and choose from the information available and apply what they've read to the care of their patients.

This book isn't about theory, although I certainly touch upon it frequently. It is about what works. I've had forty years of treating nothing but overweight patients, hundreds of thousands of them in the United States and in foreign countries, and I've certainly seen what works and what doesn't work. This book is about a method of uncovering one specific and frequent cause of overweight, a cause that is more often overlooked than discovered. It is also about how to treat that problem properly after it is discovered. As a bonus, this book is also about how to lose weight, no matter what caused the weight gain.

My methods are practical. They've worked for me and my patients. I know they will work for you.

IS YOUR THYROID MAKING YOU FAT?

1

But Doctor, I'm Telling the Truth

My patient looks troubled.

"I don't care what that doctor says, there has to be something wrong with my metabolism."

She's one of today's new patients. Her name is Marie. We've just met. She doesn't hesitate to tell me of her dissatisfaction with the last doctor she saw. I gather that her former doctor thinks she just eats too much.

"He said the tests showed that my thyroid was just fine. I followed his diet but it was just like all the others. It didn't work. I just want to be thin. What's wrong with me?"

Her words and her manner don't startle me. I've heard such words spoken too many times in the past. I truly sympathize, but at the same time I'm impatient. There's work to be done. I've a lot of questions to ask. I will do an examination. Then there will be much explaining.

Clearly Marie wants to vent her feelings, and it may be doing her good. From experience with many others, I know those feelings. At this point, I can see that she will repeat her complaint for emphasis, but I don't want to be impolite, so I let her go on. And she does.

There's no complaint I've heard more frequently during that most important first patient visit than what Marie has just expressed. Her monologue is so typical that after the first few words I could have completed her remarks. In the last thirty-eight years, I've had literally thousands of patients voice that same complaint. Of course, they aren't all as bold as this patient. They don't all blame their former doctors. They do express this same discontent, but they phrase it in many different ways:

"I don't understand why I'm so fat; I eat very little."

"I've had my thyroid tested. There's nothing wrong. Why can't I lose weight?"

"Will you give me something to burn up this fat? Nothing seems to work."

"Maybe I have a thyroid problem or something."

"No matter what I do, it won't come off."

Let's make it clear why they're telling this to me in the first place. It is because I specialize in treating overweight problems. In my medical practice, those are the only kinds of patients I see. I don't accept those whose complaint is a sore throat, a broken arm, a nasty rash, or a nose that needs to be reshaped. For forty years, I've limited myself to helping people whose ailment is an excess of fat. My experience has been acquired from hundreds of thousands of overweight patients. (I've truly lost count.)

True, a formidable number of my new patients do admit to major indiscretions. "I eat like a pig" isn't that infrequent. Marie is clearly not in that camp.

She has come to me because she has an acquaintance who seems to have undergone some sort of metamorphosis. Her friend, a once pudgy, dull, couch potato, has a new svelte figure and radiates an astounding personality change. She's given up her menial employment and is going to school to learn court reporting.

Marie knows that her friend has been my patient for a while and that I must have had something to do with that transformation. She believes that the effect of the diet I prescribed for the lady was to reduce her weight and that all the other benefits were derived from some newfound confidence. Her remade friend is now proud of her body and has acquired a self-image that causes her to regard the world as her personal oyster.

She's wrong about her friend in a lot of ways.

First of all, it isn't diet alone that is responsible for the drastic improvement in the friend's shape. And it isn't newfound confidence that makes that lady get up and go. It is the medication I prescribed for her previously undiscovered ailment that is responsible for all the changes. Taking that medication, she would have emerged from hibernation even if she hadn't been fat and lost weight. Her friend has hypothyroidism.

Marie clearly doesn't know the whole story. She's hoping I have some sort of magic diet that will finally get the weight off of her. Unlike her friend, she doesn't need her psyche altered. She has enough motivation to do things and she would do them if she weren't so tired all the time. Of course, she blames that on the extra weight she is carrying.

She isn't going to find a magic diet at my office. She has already been on too many diets. She's hostile toward her last doctor because his diet didn't work. She followed it faithfully for almost a month and lost barely four pounds. At that rate it would take her forever to get thin. He didn't seem to listen to her when she told him that she loses poorly even on the strictest of diets.

Now she's trying again. What she's telling me is that there's something wrong with the way she handles food. It's her "metabolism or something." I sense that she isn't sure of this. After all, the last doctor spent a fair amount of her money at the medical laboratory and proved to her that there's nothing wrong with her metabolism. He said that her thyroid was fine and then explained to her that "thyroid" and "metabolism" were sort of the same thing. In making his explanation, he used such mysterious terms as TSH and T3 and T4. Who can argue when such scientific proof is presented? Does any ordinary mortal dare question TSH, T3, and T4?

Like Marie, at least half of my new patients believe that something has gone wrong inside of them. They declare that, given their eating habits, they shouldn't be as fat as they are.

Many of these people have been to other doctors and have had various laboratory tests intended to show whether there was some sort of metabolic problem. More often than not, the tests come back with the results quite normal. The lab asserts that there's nothing wrong with this person's thyroid. This is one of the few instances in which a patient is truly disappointed to find out that the lab tests rule out some disease. Were the tests to have suggested a metabolic abnormality, the patient's own character would nicely be off the hook. That would prove that the obesity isn't from a lack of discipline or from some character flaw. It would show that the patient's metabolism was the culprit. No such luck for the lady sitting across from me.

On the basis of laboratory tests, doctors often form their opinions. The problem is that many of them have more confidence in laboratory results than in their own good sense. Too often, they ignore the basic principles they learned during their training and rely upon high-tech innovations to show them the way. If we doubt our own perceptions when they are inconsistent with the output of high-tech procedures, we increase the chance for a faulty diagnosis. Consequently, I believe that a large number of people suffer from an ailment that causes them to be overweight and that this condition isn't diagnosed, or perhaps it is even ignored, by a lot of physicians. The ailment is hypothyroidism.

It might not be possible to find another doctor in my area who has done more thyroid testing of patients than I have. After all, I have forty years under my belt and each patient during that time has had at least a potential thyroid problem. By the time I had perhaps seen my five thousandth or ten thousandth patient, I was already pretty disillusioned with the value of thyroid tests. Today, years later, I regard those tests as practically useless. This awareness was the major motivation for my writing this book.

Since my particular interest is the patient's weight and how to get her to part with the excess portion, the subject of metabolism and the thyroid gland has become my passion. The problems that are associated with an improperly functioning thyroid gland and the resulting abnormal metabolism extend way beyond weight. After all, the thyroid gland is a major controller of how we feel, how we act, how we look, and how we function.

People know I'm obsessed with my patients' weight. That's what brings the patients to me in the first place. As with any other complaint, an early step in the process of managing weight is establishing a diagnosis. When I make a correct diagnosis of hypothyroidism, the weight problem is on its way to being solved, and the fallout from this success extends far beyond the pounds that are lost.

In the course of attacking my patients' obesity, I've seen the most fortuitous "cures" you can imagine. I've been given undeserved credit for benefits I never even contemplated. I've seen a moderately obese woman who was resigned to the fact that she was sterile become pregnant in her later years. What joy! All I was trying to do was get twenty-five pounds off her. Of course, such surprises were more dramatic in those early days. Today, I've come to expect these little miracles, even though I'm really not looking for them. I focus on my patient's weight problem. Whatever else happens is medical serendipity.

I have seen years of excruciatingly painful periods disappear in a flash as if by magic.

I have seen phlegmatic, depressed individuals who could barely motivate themselves to get up in the morning suddenly become upbeat dynamos.

I have seen debilitating pain that flits from one location to another, pain that had confounded a bevy of specialists over the years, quietly depart without fanfare.

I have seen hair come back, anemia disappear, memory return, laxatives discontinued, and chronic fatigue become a bad dream.

I don't mean to suggest that I'm the only doctor who knows about all of this. Plenty has been written about the miseries of hypothyroidism. There are even quite a few doctors who specialize in the thyroid gland alone. They and I do part company when it comes to the method of determining who has the ailment and who doesn't, and to a certain extent, what to do about it when we find that it exists.

As I've said, I specialize in treating overweight problems. Because I've seen so many patients over the years, I've developed some very definite and perhaps unique opinions on the subject. In the course of treating thousands of patients, one may change his opinion about ideas that he had previously believed to be incontrovertible.

It is my belief that when it comes to diagnosing problems involving metabolism, the laboratory not only fails us, it even gives us deceptive information about the patient. As a result, many of the patients who consult me have been told that their metabolisms are normal even though they display many of the signs and symptoms of a low metabolism.

The signs and symptoms of hypothyroidism are well known to most doctors. The subject has hardly been ignored in the literature that doctors read. I too read the literature. I'm sure that many doctors intuitively consider hypothyroidism when the patient gives them a history of her complaint. When my own intuition suggests to me that a patient has this affliction, I would naturally like some corroborating evidence. This is the point where doctors turn to the laboratory for help. The laboratory could supply the information that would confirm the diagnosis, but the fact is that it doesn't. I've come to mistrust the laboratory when it comes to the thyroid. Where, then, can I turn for help?

Years ago we had machines that were supposed to help us medical men with metabolic testing. I did thousands of basal metabolism tests with one of these machines, but I always regarded the results as suspect. There was another curious gadget that tested the response time of the Achilles tendon reflex in the ankle. It was an attempt to measure the known connection between the speed of our reflexes and thyroid function. I can still see that look the patient got when my nurse tapped her foot with a rubber hammer. Both of these machines were eventually discredited and yet as I look back, as imprecise as they were, they were probably more reliable than today's lab when it comes to hypothyroidism.

I haven't given up on the laboratory approach, but the search for adequate laboratory tests of thyroid function must continue.

In the 1970s there was a doctor who wrote on the subject. He also mistrusted the laboratory. He had great confidence in a test that he himself had developed. It was simple and easy to perform. Observing that those with hypothyroidism seemed to have a low body temperature, his patients were required to use the thermometer to help establish the diagnosis. I agree that the method has some value, but body temperature can be quite variable for a variety of reasons. I didn't feel that his test by itself could be relied upon as definitive.

Over the years, my own test evolved. Like so many nice discoveries, it was right "under my nose" all the time. It isn't as though one day I decided to invent a test for hypothyroidism. For a long time I had been aware that the inconsistency between what some people weighed and what they actually ate pointed in the direction of hypothyroidism. This knowledge, combined with other factors I observed in the patient, would lead me to make the diagnosis. What gradually emerged was a step-by-step approach to organizing that information so it would serve as a test applicable to all patients. With the testing method I now use, I feel I have at least a 90 percent chance of diagnosing hypothyroidism correctly. What's more, now you can actually do this on yourself, and in a later chapter I'm going to show you exactly how to do it. Stay calm. I'm not going to ask you to puncture yourself or to cause yourself any discomfort. You're going to be asked to eat certain things and to jot down some numbers. When you've completed the task, I believe that you will have a better idea of the state of your metabolism than you might receive from any medical laboratory.

The tests you will be performing will be the same tests that I use every day on my own patients. Whether your thyroid is at fault or not is information that could be invaluable to you if you've had difficulty losing weight, but the benefits could also extend far beyond simply regulating your weight. After you've done the testing, I shall instruct you as to what to do with that information. A low metabolism is correctable and reversible, but that will require the assistance of an attentive physician. I'm going to help you get that information to your doctor or help you find a sympathetic doctor.

If you learn that your thyroid is normal, and you have a weight problem, the testing will still be of value. You need to know that it is normal so that you may settle down to a serious diet with the confidence that it will certainly work.

Hypothyroidism is the medical term that is applied to an underactive thyroid, a gland that doesn't secrete sufficient hormone to allow the body to function normally. In many cases but not quite all, hypothyroidism results in an excess of weight. However, there are a host of other conditions and symptoms that also result from low thyroid function. Many who suffer from excessive fatigue are mistakenly told that they have chronic fatigue syndrome. A sizable number of women going through complicated and expensive treatment to facilitate pregnancy might have immediate success if their underactive thyroid glands were properly treated. Likewise, many menstrual abnormalities are the result of low thyroid function. Psychological problems are another manifestation of hypothyroidism. In general, a hypothyroid patient who receives proper treatment can experience an across-the-board improvement in her general sense of well-being.

For whatever reason, and the reason is often the laboratory, many physicians seem to go off in other directions when patients present themselves with the characteristic signs and symptoms of hypothyroidism. An October 1996 article in *McCall's* magazine, "The Disease Doctors Miss," did a good job of explaining this phenomenon. It listed many of the symptoms that accompany hypothyroidism, and it was an appeal to the reader to prod her doctor into delving into the problem. This book has essentially the same general purpose, but it also invites you, the reader, and perhaps the victim, to take a very active role in determining whether you have a metabolic or thyroid problem.

Doctors particularly seem to ignore the patient's weight as a significant sign of hypothyroidism. This is probably because of the general tendency of the literature to downplay metabolic problems as the cause of obesity.

Of the many systems I could use to categorize my overweight patients, the simplest would place each of them in one of two categories:

1. Those who eat too much.
2. Those who don't eat too much.

As simple as that sounds, it isn't. In a sense, they all eat too much. But too much for what? The answer is too much for one's body to maintain its weight. One patient might think she eats only one-third the calories her best friend eats, but it is still too much because she's overweight and her friend isn't. If the standard by which "too much" is to be judged is the amount necessary not to create obesity, then everyone who is obese eats too much.

But "too much" may not be that much at all. I'm sure you know that each of us requires a somewhat different amount of food to maintain our respective weights. In some instances the variations among us are impressive. That is the essence of the differences in metabolism among various individuals of similar size. We do seem to burn up our calories at different rates.

When the body fails to burn sufficient calories, I choose to define that condition as hypothyroidism. The trouble is that no one has yet invented a simple gauge that we can attach to ourselves that will read out how many calories we're burning at a particular moment. Until such a device comes along, we're forced to infer how many calories we burn from some rather unreliable tables.

The questions of how many calories we need, how many we eat and how many we should eat, how many calories we burn and how many we should burn, have occupied me for a long time.

When I find someone who is out of kilter with what should be, I know I'm dealing with a thyroid problem.

The thyroid gland is located in the front of your neck below your Adam's apple, and normally it takes very trained fingers to feel it. If you do feel it easily, or, more important, if your doctor feels it, it could mean that there's a problem there. If it is readily felt, then it is probably enlarged, and that could mean one of various abnormalities. If what your doctor feels are lumps or nodules, it is mandatory that you undergo further studies. But that isn't the subject of this book. A generally enlarged thyroid gland could mean an underactive thyroid gland. Let's leave it at that.

This little gland is terribly important to your welfare. Let's examine what it does and what happens when it doesn't do what it is supposed to do.

Since the thyroid gland supplies a couple of hormones that regulate our metabolic processes, abnormalities of the gland's function are present with both overproduction of the hormones and underproduction. What is interesting and yet troublesome is that some of the symptoms of both conditions can be remarkably similar. Fortunately other symptoms aren't, and that tends to differentiate clearly between the two. We generally speak of overproduction of hormones as producing *hyperthyroidism,* a serious condition where bodily processes are speeded up. The typical hyperthyroid individual is the nervous irritable individual who seems "keyed up." Everything from eye problems to severe heart problems may accompany hyperthyroidism. The hyperthyroid sufferer is generally not overweight, and we shall not delve further into that condition.

Of course, there are a number of other diseases of the thyroid gland. There are what are known as autoimmune diseases, where one's own body attacks itself, and in this case the attack is on one's own thyroid gland. One of these is Graves' disease, a condition that got a lot of press when it was revealed that both President Bush and Mrs. Bush suffered from it. There are cancers of the thyroid and there are various nodules that can form and cause trouble. Everyone knows someone or has seen people with "goiter," which is extreme enlargement of the thyroid, usually but not always caused by too much thyroid hormone.

As I've pointed out, it is the underproduction of thyroid hormone that will concern us within these pages. More symptoms can be attributed to this single ailment than to virtually any other in the entire medical repertoire. Soon we shall review what they are. Perhaps in an effort to confound us, the disease usually displays only a few for each individual. Yet different individuals with the ailment may have virtually no symptoms in common with one another. This makes diagnosis very confusing for the doctor, and it is easy to go off in the wrong direction, suspecting other ailments.

The hyperthyroid patient often appears to be a bundle of energy; the hypothyroid one is the opposite. Slow movement, depression, and apathy are some of the qualities that are readily noticeable. In females, infertility and various menstrual abnormalities are common. The person may often feel cold (and actually may be cold!). The skin is dry, the hair lifeless, the cholesterol elevated, and, of more interest, obesity is often present. When you put these things together, you can almost bet that this is someone who has repeatedly tried to lose weight and failed.

If you are one of those for whom the diagnosis of hypothyroidism has already been correctly established, there may be real benefit in concentrating on Chapter 7, "Natural or Synthetic Treatment?," which deals with the medications used for treating hypothyroidism. Here again I'm at odds with the status quo. I believe that the drugs in standard use today for this malady aren't the best choice. I will tell you why my experience has brought me to that conclusion. It may be an uphill battle trying to convince your doctor that another approach might be better, but it is worth the attempt.

You will come across Chapter 15, which is intended to be read by your doctor. It is not strictly just for him or her. I won't mind if you choose to read it. It is essentially a condensation of what is contained in the rest of the book. It is included in the hope that you can convince your doctor to consider seriously what I have learned from my experience with these thousands of patients. I expect that there will be resistance on the part of the doctors who tend to reject ideas that don't come from their customary sources. Old habits die hard. If you can get your doctor to contact me, I will endeavor to convince him. I will even keep a list of those physicians who are willing to embrace what we know to be true. I will make the list available to readers who would like the information.

Because those who treat thyroid problems are so influenced by the dictates of the ivory-tower authorities who have ordained a rather monolithic approach to hypothyroidism, you may expect to hear, perhaps in the media, that what I have dared to include in this book is akin to heresy. I've preempted my critics by becoming my own critic, in a sense. I know what the criticism will be, and so I've constructed an imaginary conversation between one such expert and me. The debate ensues in Chapter 16, "Debating My Position."

Let's get started.

2

Hypothyroidism, the Greater Imitator

This book is about hypothyroidism, how it interferes with weight loss, and how it can be remedied.

Does this patient have hypothyroidism? That's the first thing that comes to mind when I glance at my new patient. After forty years of viewing these overweight individuals, I have concluded that for perhaps one-fourth of them, the answer to that question will turn out to be yes. I've no reason to believe that a cross section of my patient population is much different from one of the general population, and therefore I must conclude that about one-fourth of those who are overweight suffer from some degree of hypothyroidism. This is a startling assertion, one that will probably cause your family doctor's eyebrows to elevate.

Medical textbooks and articles will disagree with my numbers. You may read various estimates as to the prevalence of hypothyroidism, and my guess is that the estimates will generally be below 5 percent of the population. I believe that the percentage of the population suffering from hypothyroidism is at least twice that. Why does Dr. Siegal believe this? I can only blame it upon my experience with thousands of patients over the years. The disparity is probably the result of my unique definition of hypothyroidism. If other authorities are rather united in the 5 percent figure and I maintain that it is at least twice that, both sides may be correct if we accept that there can be more than one definition of the ailment.

My definition is based on the kind of grass-roots logic that seems to come with age and experience. I adhere to the kind of thinking that believes that if it looks like a horse, it probably is a horse. Fortunately, the word *probably* gives me leeway if it were to become necessary for me to wriggle out of such a statement.

As a doctor, it's not hard to come up with a definition for a disease, particularly a new disease. You simply listen to the patients' complaints, look them over, do some lab tests or X rays, and then declare, "These patients have Siegal's disease." And who can dispute that? The task becomes more difficult when some other doctor has already defined Siegal's disease differently. I can hear him now: "How dare this upstart attempt to redefine my disease!"

In the end, this should not turn out to be some sort of useless word game. What counts is whether the definition of the ailment contributes to helping the patient with that particular problem. I will make a strong case for the assertion that my definition of hypothyroidism does just that.

Before we get to my definition of hypothyroidism, we will have to get to the meaning of some other words that will help you to understand hypothyroidism.

Endocrine Glands

These are rather miniature chemical manufacturing devices positioned at various locations in your body. They are sometimes called ductless glands because they discharge their chemicals (hormones) directly into the bloodstream. Other glands distribute what they produce through small tubes called ducts. An example of the latter are the several sets of salivary glands that are responsible for keeping the inside of your mouth wet.

The thyroid gland is one of the endocrine glands. It sends its products directly into the bloodstream. The pituitary gland and the adrenal glands are other familiar examples of endocrine glands. Each of these glands produces its own unique chemical or chemicals that are needed to affect various processes in the body.

Hormones

The chemicals produced by the endocrine glands are called hormones. Some glands normally produce more than one hormone. These powerful chemicals function as regulators of important body processes. For example, in females, the menstrual cycle is under the control of various hormones secreted by the endocrine glands known as ovaries, as well as by other glands. Repeatedly in this book, I shall refer to the particular hormones that are secreted by the thyroid gland.

Pharmaceutical companies manufacture a variety of hormone look-alikes. Birth-control pills that simulate the functions of the hormones of the ovaries are an example. We shall pay particular attention to the attempts that have been made to simulate the thyroid hormones.

Occasionally, the actual hormones are removed from the endocrine glands of animals and are used in human medicine. Before synthetic thyroid hormones were introduced in the 1950s, many people were treated with thyroid hormone that came directly from cows and hogs. Many doctors who had prescribed these could argue that animal-derived thyroid hormone was a quite satisfactory replacement when one's own hormone production was inadequate.

The Thyroid Gland

If we were to rate the various endocrine glands as to relative importance, most authorities would probably put the pituitary gland at the top of the list. Not only does it have a prestigious location, attached to the brain, but it functions largely to regulate other endocrine glands. When its hormones reach other endocrine glands, it often causes those glands to secrete their own hormones. For this reason, the pituitary is often referred to as the Master Gland. One of the glands that is controlled by the pituitary gland is the thyroid gland.

The runner-up in the gland importance competition would undoubtedly be the thyroid gland. The body processes affected by its hormones are very many and diverse. The thyroid gland in turn controls the functions of other glands. The entire endocrine system is a complex interaction of these glands and their hormones. The ultimate purpose is to keep the human machine running properly. When the thyroid gland malfunctions, the entire body is thrown into a chaotic disequilibrium.

Your thyroid gland is located in front of the lower part of your neck. If you press your index finger into the very bottom of your neck in the front, you will find a distinct notch in the bone below. This is the top of a bone called the sternum, and the notch should distinctly cradle your finger. The next two or three inches above the notch to the left and the right is occupied by your thyroid gland. It actually has two parts, one on either side. Don't be concerned if you can't feel it. If the gland is normal in size, it is difficult to find. If it is enlarged, you may feel it; it has the consistency of a ripe peach. If you have considerable fat in this area, you will probably not be able to differentiate the gland from the surrounding fat. It is really not very important that you find your thyroid gland or even feel it. Let's leave that to your doctor. I was obliged to locate it for you. After all, if you're going to read a book about your thyroid gland, you should at least know where it is.

What It Does

The thyroid gland has many functions, but the one I shall give the most attention to is how it controls the rate at which your body uses energy. If that sentence seems somewhat mysterious, I could perhaps clarify it by making substitutions for some of the words. I could replace "the rate at which" with "how fast." "Energy" could be "calories" or even "food." I could use the time-worn analogy of the automobile. Your body is the car and it needs fuel to power the engine. The fuel could come from the outside—in other words, your food. But your food must first be converted into a more refined type of fuel before your engine can utilize it. Your fuel could also come from your storage tank, that layer of fat you would like to be rid of. But even that must be converted into a different form before it can be "burned."

I have said that the thyroid controls how fast the fuel is used. A better explanation is that it controls how much fuel is needed to perform a particular task. In an automobile, the task is to move some passengers from Point A to Point B. Of course, a heavier car or a heavier load will need more fuel. So will a heavier body or one that is performing a more strenuous task. There is a distinction between our objectives when we compare our bodies with our cars.

With automobiles, fuel efficiency is what we strive for. Let's get the most miles per gallon. The auto industry, if we're to believe its spokespeople, is on a constant campaign to improve fuel efficiency, to build cars that will get more miles to the gallon. Strangely enough, those who are overweight would like to achieve the opposite effect. What they would hope for and what they probably don't have is a real gas burner. They want a very inefficient engine that will guzzle fuel. Of course, the fuel you want to waste is your stored fuel, your fat. If there is a day when you're too busy to eat, you will have to dip into your stored fat to supply energy to your engine. You would probably hope that your body would somehow use twice that amount of fuel (energy, calories) that day. At the same time, you would probably wish for your actual car to get twice the mileage from its fuel.

Your thyroid gland in secreting its hormones regulates this use of fuel by your body. If it malfunctions by secreting too little hormone, your body processes slow down. That is another way of saying that you use less fuel. This is one explanation for why some people weigh more than they should. There are other possibilities. It is quite possible that the gland doesn't malfunction but some other mechanism does, but the result is the same. If the targets of the thyroid hormone, the cells that actually carry out the fuel consumption, somehow don't interpret the stimulating effect of the thyroid hormone, fuel consumption doesn't increase. As I've indicated, the effect is the same: less fuel consumption. The solution to the problem is also the same, but how this problem can be solved will come later.

Part of my definition of hypothyroidism is derived from this concept. If the secretion of thyroid hormone isn't sufficient to cause the body to burn calories at a normal rate, it is hypothyroidism. If a "normal" amount of thyroid hormone is secreted but it doesn't achieve the calorie-consuming effect it should, we essentially have the same problem, and I still define it as hypothyroidism. The *hypo-* prefix to a medical term means "low" or "not enough." The *hyper-* prefix means just the opposite. There is indeed a *hyperthyroidism,* a condition in which too many calories are consumed for a given task.

The abnormal burning of calories is the component of hypothyroidism that may generate the most interest, but there are many more signs and symptoms. There are so many and they affect so many diverse bodily systems that it is easy to confuse hypothyroidism with a multitude of other diseases. Even though doctors have nicknamed another disease, syphilis, the "great imitator" because its many manifestations can suggest a variety of other ailments, hypothyroidism may well be an even greater imitator. Presently, I shall go into an exploration of many of the conditions that may accompany hypothyroidism. What often makes the diagnosis difficult for the physician is the fact that although a variety of signs and symptoms is possible, in reality, the usual sufferer displays a relatively small number of them. You can see how confusing the diagnostic task could be. One patient could have three of the signs of hypothyroidism while another has three entirely different signs, yet they both have hypothyroidism. This, coupled with what I believe is a basic flaw in current theory regarding thyroid hormones, often leads to a missed diagnosis.

There is one symptom that is always present, and that is the abnormal consumption of calories. But this is an invisible symptom. You can't see it or feel that it is there. It operates silently and quite undercover. There are some who may dispute my statement that it is always present, but I declare it with the assurance that comes from viewing thousands of patients over many years. This is the common denominator of hypothyroidism, and this fact forms the basis of the MFI test that will be described later. This quirk of hypothyroidism is what enables me to single out those afflicted, often those who have previously been told there is nothing wrong with their thyroid gland.

Those who would dispute what I've just said will probably be quick to ask, "If that is true, why aren't all of those with hypothyroidism overweight?" That is indeed a good question, but it's one that isn't too difficult to answer. In order for anyone to become overweight, he or she must consume more calories than his or her body requires to function normally. The excess food (calories) is stored as fat. The hypothyroid patient who eats a *normal* quantity of food over a period of time will gain weight because his or her usage of calories is less than it should be. But a hypothyroid individual who eats *less* than a normal quantity of food may not gain. Remember, there are those who eat excessively, those who eat rather normally, and others who eat fewer calories than are generally needed to maintain a fixed weight, and this is irrespective of their thyroid function. Those who eat minimally may maintain their weight on a diet that would cause "normal" individuals to lose weight. In other words, the hypothyroid individual may still eat so little that the amount consumed is simply not enough to cause weight gain in spite of the low rate of metabolism.

Thyroid Hormone Production

Research scientists tell us that the production of thyroid hormones by the thyroid gland is stimulated by another hormone from the pituitary gland. This hormone, thyroid stimulating hormone, is usually referred to as TSH. Its production is in turn triggered by yet another hormone. An important constituent of the thyroid hormones is iodine. The thyroid gland uses iodine found in the diet to manufacture its two main substances, which I shall call by their abbreviated names, T3 and T4. The gland actually produces about four times as much T4 as T3, but since the latter is much more potent, the net effect is that they each contribute about the same amount to the metabolic effect.

There are areas of the world where iodine in the food supply is deficient, and in these areas thyroid disease is far more prevalent. In the United States, this is particularly true around the Great Lakes. In Europe, Switzerland is the most noteworthy for this. The use of salt containing iodine (iodized salt) is widespread around the world, and this is probably a major factor in preventing the problem.

A frequent result of insufficient intake of iodine is goiter, which is simply an enlarged thyroid gland. There are various types of goiter, and goiter can even be caused by an excessive intake of iodine. It isn't difficult to spot individuals who have this enlargement at the base of their necks.

It is believed that T3 is actually the hormone that works directly upon the body's cells, but the cells have the ability to convert T4 into T3. Of course, before any of these hormones, TSH, T3, or T4, can do their work, they must be transported to the work site, and they are carried to these sites by the blood. Scientists have developed tests to detect the amounts of these hormones in the patient's blood, and it is logical that doctors use these tests in order to determine the status of an individual's thyroid function. From the blood levels of these substances, the diagnosis of an underactive (or an overactive) thyroid is made. In fact, doctors rely heavily upon these test results. They are used everywhere. They are the current basis for the diagnosis of hypothyroidism.

The Causes of Hypothyroidism

The causes of most cases of hypothyroidism are unknown, although hereditary factors are certainly involved. It may skip generations. Other causes are man-made. It may result from other types of therapy. For example, irradiating the thyroid gland is a common treatment for an overactive gland (hyperthyroidism), and it generally results in some degree of underactivity. The surgical removal of a major portion of the gland would have the same result. Exposure to accidental radiation such as what happened at Chernobyl is another. The lithium drugs used to treat depression may also initiate hypothyroidism.

The vast majority of patients I see have no clear-cut cause that can be detected. If heredity is important, it isn't easily traced. Previous cases in a family often went undetected. I have my suspicions as to what some of the causes might be. I think it is curious that I see more cases in women who have had recent pregnancies than in those who have never been pregnant. Patients with hypothyroidism will often describe a recent emotional shock, or their lives may be particularly stressful.

Steroid drugs (such as prednisone or hydrocortisone) are often used to treat inflammation, allergy, and other conditions and are widely prescribed by doctors. Although these medications seem to work miracles in relieving many symptoms, there has always been controversy over their use or their overuse. I think it is more than coincidence that many of my hypothyroid patients have at some time or another had a course of steroid treatment.

There are even those cases where one's own body is the villain. One of these is the autoimmune disease Hashimoto's thyroiditis (named for its Japanese discoverer), in which substances in one's own blood attack the thyroid gland and destroy much of its functionality. Fortunately, this disease responds to treatment much like other forms of hypothyroidism.

Other Thyroid Disorders

The thyroid gland can also be the site of various other medical problems, but it is beyond the scope of this book to examine them in detail. Just as hypothyroidism is characterized by insufficient amounts or effects of thyroid hormone, there may also be an over-abundance of the hormone. As I have mentioned, this condition is called hyperthyroidism. The symptoms are quite different from hypothyroidism. As you might expect, they are somewhat the opposite. Even though this individual burns calories at a rate higher than normal, that effect can be overcome by eating excessively, and the individual may end up overweight. Usually those afflicted are quite thin, but don't be too quick to envy those souls. Their problem has the potential of being even more serious.

Hyperthyroidism is relatively common and perhaps missed less often by doctors than hypothyroidism. While one form of hyperthyroidism, Graves' disease, attacked President and Mrs. Bush, it was reported by the press that even the White House dog suffered from a thyroid disorder. This sent people scurrying to test the water supply at their residence, but they apparently came up with a blank. Since Graves' disease is common, this was probably just an unusual coincidence.

Like other body parts, the thyroid may play host to a variety of tumors and cancers. I don't treat these conditions. When they are suspected, the patient is referred to the appropriate specialist. If your interest in the thyroid gland goes beyond hypothyroidism, I would recommend some of the books listed in Appendix H.

Signs and Symptoms of Hypothyroidism

I have mentioned that the signs and symptoms of hypothyroidism are many, yet a particular individual may have but a few. What follows is a list, which may not be complete, since new items seem to be added to the list constantly. You might conclude that anyone perusing this list might come to the conclusion that he or she is afflicted, and that is exactly why the ailment is so often missed. Who doesn't have some of these? Yet every case of constipation isn't hypothyroidism. Let's look at the list. I've placed the symptoms in alphabetical order.

Anemia
Brittle nails
Cold intolerance
Constipation
Depression
Dry or coarse hair
Dry skin
Fatigue
Hair loss
Headaches
Hoarse voice
Impotence
Infertility
Irritability
Low body temperature
Memory loss
Menstrual pain and other abnormalities
Miscarriages
Muscle pain or cramps
Overweight
Palpitations
Puffy facial features
Sleeping excessively
Slow pulse
Weakness

I'm sure that everyone who reads this list can identify with something on it. That doesn't make the diagnosis of hypothyroidism. Were there not some common factor that all hypothyroid victims possessed, the list would not be that helpful in diagnosing the ailment. Current thinking in most of the medical community is that the common factor is none of the above, but rather certain abnormal results obtained from blood tests. Experience has caused me to disagree. I believe that a far more reliable test is based on the common factor of low metabolic rate, the subnormal utilization of stored calories. I shall expand on this in the chapters to come, and you will learn how you can do a self-test of your own metabolic rate.

I Want to Lose Weight

A patient doesn't consult me because of the usual symptoms of hypothyroidism such as hair loss, or depression, or because she hasn't been able to become pregnant. She is there because she has heard that I can help her to lose weight. If she has any of the symptoms from the above list, she probably has not connected them with her weight problem. To learn more about them, I must pry the information out of her. In the course of a medical history you learn a lot if you ask a lot of questions. Although I'm always looking for hypothyroidism, the physical appearance of a particular patient may be quite contrary to the stereotype for this ailment, and I relax my vigil. The right answers to a few questions can definitely put me back on the right track.

A statement that never fails to attract my attention is "No matter what I do, I can't lose weight," or something similar. "I really don't overeat" will also start the wheels turning. "The last doctor said there is nothing wrong with my thyroid" is particularly significant. It tells me that someone at least suspected hypothyroidism, either the doctor or the patient. If neither had entertained the idea, there would have been no point in the doctor making that assertion.

Now armed with a real suspicion, I'm ready for some further corroborating evidence: "Yes, my hair is very dry." "I have these

aches and pains and no one can find out what's wrong with me."
"I've had this raspy voice ever since my pregnancy."

This is all it takes for me to launch the test. It is actually what I refer to as the determination of the patient's Metabolic Function Index. It is my invention, so I had to give it a name. MFI is a lot easier to say, so that is what I will call it in these pages.

It will take about four weeks until I know what the MFI is for this patient, and until then she will be treated much as any other patient who comes to lose weight: a diet, counseling, perhaps medication to help with hunger, and perhaps treatment for some unrelated condition. If and when I find that she has a subnormal MFI, her treatment routine will change.

I don't mean to suggest that only suspicious cases are tested. In a sense, every patient is tested. An inadequate weight loss in four weeks coupled with a patient who has seriously complied with her instructions is a real red flag for hypothyroidism. For the patient who is under suspicion, I probably work harder to impress upon her the necessity for complying during this first month. I tell her that if she doesn't deviate from the diet, I (and she) will have valuable information that could serve her well in the future.

The prospect that she will once and for all learn why she cannot lose weight combined with the expectation that the problem can be corrected can be a powerful motive for cooperation. In this case cooperation means adhering strictly to a particular diet for four solid weeks. It isn't very hard to convince a patient that this exercise is worth the effort.

If you have truly had difficulty in losing weight, or if you're overweight and believe that the calories you consume don't account for it, it would be to your advantage to take the test in Chapter 12. If you have several of the signs and symptoms listed above, this should underline your need to know. You should take the test particularly if you have already had blood tests that supposedly ruled out a thyroid problem. No effort in obtaining valuable information about yourself is ever wasted.

Let's not be too quick to jump to conclusions. Yes, it may be your impression that you don't lose weight as you should. You may also have a few of the listed symptoms. That is the starting point for putting your curiosity to good use. I will give you the means to really find out.

Hypothyroidism is treatable, and when it is treated, weight loss suddenly becomes easier and most of its other manifestations are reversed.

Summing Up

- Hypothyroidism is more widespread than it is generally believed to be.
- The thyroid gland controls the rate at which we use energy.
- Hypothyroidism has many different signs and symptoms, but a particular sufferer may only have a very few.
- Hypothyroidism is characterized by the slow burning of calories.
- There is a home test that one can perform based on calorie consumption that can show the presence or the absence of hypothyroidism.

3

Disenchantment with the Laboratory

Patients who come to me for help have generally sought help before from other doctors, so-called clinics, or organizations. It is uncommon for me to see a new patient who has never attempted to lose weight with some outside help. Occasionally the help was from a magazine article or a diet book, but much more frequently it was through some more structured system.

There are the "clinics" that have no medical connection that give dietary advice and usually accompany their instructions with mandatory prepared meals that are sold to the client. There are the organizations that emphasize group enthusiasm (or shame) along with their diets. Any of these can work reasonably well if the client is well motivated and doesn't want to waste her money. In the long term they usually fail, since the client doesn't maintain whatever weight is achieved, and that is true for most methods.

Many people go to doctors to lose weight. Some of the best results as well as some of the worst seem to come from physicians. Many doctors take a real personal interest in their dieting patients, and some patients do perform admirably under their scrutiny. Unfortunately, there are also doctors who write a prescription for three months' worth of appetite suppressants and then tear a sheet off of a pad of diets, seeing the patient off with instructions to behave for the next three months. The success rate there is infinitesimal.

From talking to colleagues over the years and from listening to lecturers at seminars, I have the distinct impression that for many physicians, from that first moment an overweight patient walks through the door, there is the presumption, a well-entrenched mind-set, that she is a glutton and that, consistent with human nature, she will deny the fact that she is such. Thus, when she declares the proverbial "I eat like a bird," the classic cartoon balloon appears above the doctor's head, illustrating what is in his mind: The bird, a vulture, is flying off to its feast, its talons locked onto a substantial hog.

The fact is that in this arena, and perhaps others (or perhaps in no other), doctors mistrust the patient's honesty. What's more, the patient senses that the doctor doesn't believe her. I often see this in the uncomfortable way a patient informs me that she doesn't overeat. She isn't relaxed in telling me this, not because she is lying, but because she expects me to think she is lying. It isn't unusual for a lady to bring her husband into the treatment room with her. It's clear that he is there as a character witness to vouch for her honesty. ("Honest, Doc. She really doesn't eat.")

Nonetheless, disregarding their own preconceived notions, many physicians address the possibility of hypothyroidism by ordering tests that purport to supply the answers. Once this is done, the test results seem to become the end in themselves rather than a step along the way.

"Your thyroid gland tests normal. You really should lose that weight. I'm going to give you a diet. . . ."

This all concerns a mythical doctor and his mythical patient. Allow me to expand on the mythical discussion:

"But, Doctor, I've tried low-calorie diets and they don't work.

I told you how tired I am. I read this article in a magazine that said my weight problem and my fatigue could be due to—"

"Yes, we can't ignore that fatigue. I'm going to order some additional tests to try to rule out certain ailments. . . ."

And so it goes. This scenario has repeatedly been played out to me by my patients.

I believe our doctor has dropped the ball. Infectious mononucleosis should not be at the top of his agenda. Had he not been so certain that his patient was lying from the beginning, he might have entertained the idea that the lab made a mistake. Laboratories do make mistakes. If this patient's lab work came back with a blood glucose reading of 275, he would probably have asked her to repeat the test before he pronounced her a diabetic. But since the thyroid results rubber-stamped what he believed from the onset, he had no difficulty in dismissing her protestations.

I must point out that I use the laboratory constantly in acquiring information about the states of my patients' health. Most laboratory tests are really quite reliable. But not all.

I have virtually no confidence in the results of laboratory thyroid testing.

I suspect that people have been burned at the stake for uttering less blasphemous sentences.

I have ordered literally thousands of thyroid tests for my patients over the years. In the beginning and according to my training, I would accept the results as valuable tools to separate those overweight patients whose problem was complicated by an underactive thyroid from those with normal thyroid function.

Almost from the beginning, I would notice that some patients who professed their innocence in terms of overeating had normal thyroid values. It took a while for me to become brave enough to go against proper procedure and actually prescribe a small amount of thyroid hormone to someone who wasn't supposed to need it. On the relatively few occasions when I would do this, the patient's response to treatment was often dramatic. I'm not sure how I actually rationalized my deviation from what was considered proper. Perhaps I explained it to myself by excusing the lab for some error in technique, or by telling myself I had a patient whose blood had some mysterious quality that rendered it impossible to analyze accurately.

This began to happen more and more until I realized that although I was doing a lot of thyroid testing, I was very frequently ignoring the results. Eventually this evolved into my not bothering to run tests for which I knew I would ignore the results. I didn't do this casually. Perhaps the most disappointing aspect of the testing was that sometimes I would order a repeat test and get entirely different results. A more flagrant scenario was played out when on a few occasions I would order the tests three days in a row on the same patient and get totally diverse results. How would any doctor know which result to rely upon?

I have virtually no confidence in the results of laboratory thyroid testing. It was much easier to say that the second time after I had given my justification. I now know that if I were to use only the results of the most common thyroid tests, mainly the TSH, the T4, and the T3, I would be in the dark as to who had hypothyroidism and who didn't.

Why, then, do other doctors not feel the same way? I don't know the answer, but I can tell you that I'm mystified as to why. I'm sure that many of them have observed what I have. On several occasions I have spoken to other physicians about this, and I have had the distinct impression that a number of them have agreed with me. Their observations were similar. They recognized that the laboratory thyroid results often didn't seem to coincide with the patient's history and observations made during the physical. But that is where the scientific curiosity seemed to end. The doctors simply wrote off the discrepancy as some unexplained phenomenon and then continued to follow the old rules.

I have even had many doctors and nurses as patients over the years with whom I have discussed this. Some of them turned out to have hypothyroidism that was previously undiscovered, and they responded to treatment nicely. But I've never had the feeling that anything I had to say disturbed the status quo. If they were impressed, it didn't seem to go beyond the belief that they were unique and that my deviant treatment was applicable only in their particular case.

I'm not the first to voice such heretical statements concerning thyroid testing. Dr. Broda Barnes, in his 1976 book *Hypothy- roidism: The Unsuspected Illness* (co-authored by Lawrence Galton), expressed my same displeasure with laboratory testing. He also had treated thousands of patients and was frustrated by the lack of proper testing methods. He bemoaned the fact that science can monitor a man's heart while he's walking on the moon, but sci- entists can't develop an adequate test of thyroid function. He said,

> The efforts through the various tests to measure thyroid activity by determining the amount of the hormone stored in the gland or alternatively the amount present in the bloodstream fail to do what really counts: provide an indication of the amount of thyroid hormone avail- able and being used within cells throughout the body.

Barnes was pointing out that although the tests may indeed be accurate in determining how much thyroid hormone is in the blood at that moment, this knowledge may be useless. It is in the individual cells that the thyroid hormone does its work. If the hormone doesn't get to the cell or if the cell cannot accept or use the hormone, then it matters little how much of the substance is in the bloodstream.

Dr. Barnes actually relied upon a test of his own and although it was primitive, it was in his opinion still better than anything else around. It is a well-known fact that patients with hypothy- roidism run a lower body temperature than the rest of the popu- lation. He instructed his patients (and his readers) to take their body temperature. I would agree with him that the temperature test is worth more than the blood tests. Yet to rely upon that method suffers from the fact that many other immediate body states can alter one's body temperature. An undetected infection is an example. If I have any criticism of Dr. Barnes's method, it is that he seems to have relied on a single temperature reading to make his decision as to hypothyroidism in the patient. It would seem that multiple readings over a period of days might be more reliable. Still, anything that points us in the right direction is useful. Later you will learn how I add a variation of Barnes's temperature test to my own method.

At this point, the idea isn't so much to second-guess your doctor as it is to do a little individual homework and, based on your results, make a decision as to how to proceed. If what you've read so far has you a little suspicious that you may have some degree of hypothyroidism, a later chapter will give you the means to investigate it for yourself. There are a couple of questions you should now be asking yourself:

Do I believe that my weight is justified by the diet I eat?
Do I have some of the other signs and symptoms of hypothyroidism?

Having asked these questions and stored the information in your brain, you may now go on to learn what thyroid testing is really all about.

Before your doctor does any specific testing for thyroid problems, he will generally have done a more general series of tests designed to uncover trouble spots in a variety of the body's systems. Twenty to thirty of these tests are usually lumped together as a group by the individual laboratories and are given a name by the lab, for example, the General Profile. Not all labs choose the identical group of tests for inclusion in this general profile, but certain tests will undoubtedly be included in every lab's choice. A general profile of this type will always include tests for blood glucose (sugar), cholesterol, blood urea nitrogen, serum sodium, etc. It isn't routine for laboratories to include any specific thyroid tests in this profile. They must be ordered separately. Even though twenty or more tests are done in such a profile, the patient is generally overjoyed to learn that only one blood specimen is needed for the entire group of tests.

After your doctor has examined the results of this laboratory profile, he may then focus in on any tests that come back with abnormal results and order further, more specific tests that will target particular body systems or specific ailments. As an example, if the physician finds the blood glucose level to be elevated, he will probably choose to order a glucose tolerance test, which will give much more specific information as to the presence of diabetes.

Since thyroid tests aren't a part of this profile, before the doctor orders further thyroid testing, something in the results will probably trigger his interest. The particular test that should alert him to the possibility of hypothyroidism is an elevated level of blood cholesterol. This is a frequent finding in hypothyroidism. Sadly, I see one patient after another who has been tested by the primary-care physician, been found to have an elevated cholesterol level, and been given a prescription for one of the new and obscenely expensive cholesterol-lowering agents with the admonition to stop eating so much fat.

The prevailing standard of medical care, but in my opinion not the proper one, would dictate that our physician should have ordered the next round of tests with the objective of ruling out hypothyroidism as the cause of the elevated cholesterol. If he were to have followed current practice guidelines, he would have ordered three more tests: the T3, the T4, and the TSH.

The Standard Thyroid Tests

The T4 test in its most current form, done by radioimmunoassay, detects the amount of the thyroid hormone thyroxine (T4) circulating in the bloodstream. T4 accounts for 80 percent of the thyroid gland's production of hormones. If the blood levels of T4 are low, the theory is that the body's cells aren't getting enough of this hormone and the patient is thus suffering from hypothyroidism.

The T3 test similarly measures the amount of this other thyroid hormone found in the bloodstream. Although it accounts for only about 20 percent of the thyroid gland's production, it has a much more powerful effect, so that T4 and T3 share rather equally the total hormonal effect of the thyroid. Additionally, T3 is produced in the cells when T4 is converted into T3.

The TSH (thyroid stimulating hormone) test is generally accepted (but not by this doctor) as the most reliable screening test for overproduction or underproduction of thyroid hormones. TSH is actually a hormone of another gland, the pituitary gland, and this TSH causes the thyroid gland to secrete its hormones. The theory is that the pituitary gland recognizes an insufficient level of circulating thyroid hormones and secretes its TSH into the bloodstream. This causes the thyroid gland to secrete more hormones, T4 and T3. The pituitary gland now senses the increased production and shuts down its secretion of TSH. Thus, the two glands work together to keep the correct amount of thyroid hormones circulating.

Doctors make their diagnosis based on the blood levels of these various substances. Various combinations of high and low values for each of these tests should enable us to narrow down the site and nature of the problem. Repeatedly the literature speaks of the TSH test as the single most important tool for the diagnosis of thyroid problems.

There are even additional tests that further purport to narrow down the causes of the problem. All of this boils down to a very "scientific" organized system of diagnosing a disease that causes major inconveniences to the sufferer. It's all very nice and neat and methodical. The problem is that in the eyes of this practitioner, the method just doesn't work.

If I were to follow the "cookbook" set of rules that has been suggested by these preceding paragraphs (as I once did), my life would be a lot simpler. I would look at a few numbers on the lab reports, immediately see the problem, and respond according to an equally organized set of rules in treating (or not treating) my patient. But I can't do that.

I can't do that because I know from experience that the diagnosis of thyroid problems isn't that simple. I know that if I were to follow this accepted procedure I would miss more hypothyroidism than I would diagnose correctly. Furthermore, I would label some patients as hypothyroid when they weren't at all. It took a lot of years, a lot of patients, and a lot of thyroid tests to bring me to that conclusion. That is the purpose of this book. I want to alert you, the potential patient, as well as your doctor, not to accept the gospel of laboratory infallibility.

Is there any value at all in doing these tests? I've asked myself that question more times than I care to count. Suppose I form the impression that a particular new patient indeed has many signs that make me suspicious of hypothyroidism. Suppose I then subjected the patient to Dr. Siegal's MFI test, which I shall describe later, and it corroborates my suspicions. If I then run the "proper" thyroid tests and the results confirm that my suspicions were correct, I would be able to congratulate myself for being such a discerning doctor and I could proceed to treat my patient's hypothyroidism. If the course of treatment produced a radical improvement, i.e., the patient lost a ton of weight and virtually all of her symptoms disappeared, it would further attest to my skill as a physician.

But suppose in the above scenario I had performed the laboratory tests and the results clearly disagreed with my suspicions. Would I then act differently? Would I then say, "Everything points to hypothyroidism, but the laboratory has proven me wrong, so I must reject that idea"? Of course not. I would proceed to do exactly as I had done in the first example, perhaps leaving off the extra pat on the back. I would treat the patient for her hypothyroidism exactly as in the first example.

However, what if in this second scenario the patient didn't respond positively to treatment? I would have to accept that my judgment had been wrong and that the laboratory had been right. In practice, that hasn't happened, or, to be more exact, it has happened so seldom that I must regard it as the rare exception to the rule.

I introduced this series of hypothetical possibilities with the question of whether the lab tests have any value at all. It is clear that in my opinion they have little value, because they don't influence in any way my approach to the patient.

It isn't easy to take such an adverse position. One must question one's own judgment when it has such a minority viewpoint within a universe of supposedly competent scientists. Yet is my own personal experience not to be trusted? The laboratory has failed me. My own intuition, coupled with techniques I've yet to tell you about, has served me and my patients well. No, I must stick to my guns. There is a better way to determine who has hypothyroidism and who doesn't. You will soon learn my method. You may even learn why weight loss has been so difficult for you to achieve.

Summing Up

- Many physicians place complete confidence in the laboratory results for thyroid function, ignoring obvious symptoms in their patients.
- The laboratory cannot be relied upon when diagnosing hypothyroidism.
- An indicator of low thyroid function is lower-than-normal body temperature.
- Elevated cholesterol in the blood is a common symptom of hypothyroidism.

4

It's Not Always Overeating

Early in the medical history of each new patient I take on I ask, "What do you think is the cause of your weight problem?" As you might expect, I get a variety of responses. Sometimes the blank stare that follows suggests that my patient has never considered that there was such a thing as a cause. It is accepted that being overweight is a condition that simply exists. For those patients, speculating as to the cause isn't worth the effort. But that isn't the usual response. Without a doubt, what I hear most is "I just eat too much."

This is certainly an honest response, and it doesn't always pop out that spontaneously. I often have to dig it out. Typical of such an exchange was my initial history-taking session with Cindy, who supervised the staff of a law office:

"What do you think has caused you to be overweight?"

"Well, I've a very stressful job. I manage an office full of people and they drive me mad."

"What does that have to do with being overweight?"

"I don't have a minute to myself. I work maybe twelve hours a day. It's very stressful."

"Do you think stress makes you overweight?"

"Absolutely. If I had a more relaxed job, I don't think I would have this problem."

"Does eating have anything to do with it?"

"Of course. I have to eat what I can get. I don't have time to eat right. To top it off, the attorneys are always bringing goodies into the office. When you're hungry, it's hard to resist."

There is certainly a reluctance on my patient's part to admit that she overeats. It took several sentences before the word *eat* or *food* was even mentioned. I have concluded that people don't like to admit that they overeat. There must be some shame connected with it. They hem and haw so that they don't have to use those damning words. Still, Cindy was basically honest; she just took an oblique road to admitting that she overeats. About half of my new patients either immediately or eventually get around to confessing that they eat too much. Even then, what I hear more often is that they eat "the wrong things" rather than "too much." Cindy turned out not to have a thyroid problem; her test month resulted in an acceptable weight loss. She went on to become a model patient. Once she got into gear, she was able to resist those temptations.

A small number will explain their weight problems by indicating that obesity is a family trait. If I push them to elaborate upon how their genes contribute to weight, they will usually explain that their parents, their brothers and sisters, and assorted aunts and uncles are all obese. I try to probe deeper to see if they are pointing to a type of behavior—overeating—they learned from their relatives, or whether they are suggesting that they have inherited a metabolic problem. The latter is certainly a recognized concept. Hypothyroidism does seem to pass from one generation to the next.

The other half of my patients profess not to overeat. They express this with varying degrees of certainty: "I don't think I eat more than I should. My husband eats more than I do and he's thin." "I eat half as much as many of my friends and I'm still fatter than any of them." This half of my patient population suggests that there is a metabolic problem. They may not be clear that they are speaking of a thyroid problem, but they feel that there is *something* wrong with them.

About half of the group who believe something is wrong with them are actually wrong about that. Their problem is that they do overeat. Perhaps they just don't realize how much they do eat, or, more likely, they are nursing some sort of denial mechanism. When questioned, the facts come out and the patients often seem embarrassed. They do make a distinction between "eating" and "snacking." Eating is what you do sitting down at specific, set times. Snacking is done on the run. I've even had patients who declared they never eat a meal and therefore can't understand why they have a weight problem. They are slow to accept that all that food they've eaten apart from meals amounts to more calories than the three meals they've missed.

It is the other half of that *something-must-be-wrong* group that holds the greatest interest for me. These are the patients who truly don't overeat. It isn't unusual for me to have to elicit this information from someone who accompanies them into my office, a wife, a friend, a sister perhaps. They are sure they eat less than anyone else around them. They are also the most vocal in telling me about it. I've referred to these people earlier. They are emphatic and quite often somewhat angry. I'm not sure if this has resulted from the belief that they've been dealt the wrong cards in life or whether the stigma of excess weight has evoked undeserved disapproval from others. It is this very agitated state that works against their making their points. I expect that if these patients do have thyroid problems it would be more characteristic for them to be quite docile, and I'm always surprised to see this obvious agitation. The subject must be troubling enough for them to muster some gumption.

I estimate that about one-fourth of my patients do have some degree of hypothyroidism. This is probably at least double what is reported in the medical literature. It is hard for me to make an actual assessment of how prevalent hypothyroidism is. Remember, I see only those hypothyroid individuals who are overweight. There may be many out there who aren't overweight or perhaps are only moderately so, and they would have no reason to consult me.

There are degrees of hypothyroidism, and in the first encounter the disorder may not be obvious. In some, I can spot it before they've uttered a word. It is their characteristic puffy appearance, their slow-moving ways, their lack of enthusiasm. Yet in others I'm surprised to find that it exists. Some simply don't match the stereotype.

What is the stereotype? The textbooks describe a male or a female with puffy, dry skin, coarse hair, and a hoarse voice, who is slow to respond to questions, someone who projects the image of the couch potato. Yet I've seen hypothyroidism in individuals who had none of these characteristics. I'm not sure that there is any other ailment with such a multitude and diversity of symptoms. What confounds us doctors is the knowledge that only a fraction of these symptoms are usually present in a particular patient, and those symptoms could just as easily be associated with an entirely different ailment.

I remember a patient by the name of Jean who had a slew of hypothyroid signs and symptoms and who had had blood tests with her family doctor. She had accepted that she had a normal thyroid. She was not angry with anyone; she took it philosophically. She had so much respect for her family doctor that she couldn't bring herself to doubt him. She also knew that her meager eating habits should not have accounted for her 192 pounds. I'm not sure how she was able to rationalize this paradox in her mind. When I spoke of doing my thyroid test, she replied, "Oh no, I've really been tested. There's absolutely nothing wrong with my thyroid." Since the diet and test are the same thing, she was tested anyway. When I told her I believed she had a thyroid problem, she resisted my suggestion that she be treated for it. After a month of virtually no weight loss, she acquiesced and began to lose weight satisfactorily. She reached the goal we set and even continued to maintain her 128 pounds with the help of the thyroid hormone I had prescribed. If you were to approach her and ask her about herself, I wouldn't be surprised if she were to tell you that she has no thyroid problem.

Later I shall elaborate on what I believe to be the common denominator of hypothyroidism, the slow burning of calories. You must take care not to assume that this automatically equates to being overweight. Remember, excess weight occurs when one takes in more calories than one requires. Hypothyroid people need fewer calories. But if they are poor eaters and they don't take in more than they need, then they aren't overweight.

Hypothyroidism may be present from birth, and it is a severe problem when it exists in the newborn. Fortunately, pediatricians seem very attuned to discovering these afflicted babies, and it is my impression that in this country very few go untreated. It is the hypothyroidism that is acquired later with which I most frequently deal.

Today, I'm very attuned to spotting the potential victim, and every patient is evaluated with that possibility considered. This wasn't always the case. I have already spoken of how my methods have changed as my experience has broadened. I must admit that I cringe when I consider the number of cases I must have missed in those early years. I can remember repeated scenarios where I was completely befuddled by the patient who didn't lose weight adequately.

Back then, I was more in awe of the laws of the universe. I knew that in order for a person to lose one pound of body fat, his intake of calories had to be 3,500 calories fewer than the body needed during that period of time. I still believe this. That was the basis of my bewilderment. Cathy brought in the food diary she had meticulously kept for the preceding four weeks. Using her little calorie book, she had diligently calculated the calories in each morsel she had eaten. She had lost less than one pound over the four-week period, and her diet averaged 1,200 calories a day. That didn't add up. The charts said that Cathy needed about 2,000 calories a day just to maintain her weight. That means there was an 800-calorie deficit each day. In twenty-eight days the deficit was 22,400. That should have meant a loss of about six pounds.

She had been tested with the usual laboratory thyroid workup. The laboratory tests revealed that her thyroid hormone levels were perfect. What was wrong? Maybe her arithmetic was bad. Maybe she forgot to include that hot-fudge sundae each night at bedtime. Maybe she was just storing a lot of water and she really had lost six pounds of fat. Maybe I wrote down the wrong weight on that last visit. Maybe . . .

Of course any one of these possibilities could have explained the discrepancy. But over the years this kind of thing happened again and again with hundreds of patients (maybe thousands). It finally sank in. These "normal" patients weren't all that normal. Abnormal problems require abnormal solutions. I truly can't remember the very first time I deviated from accepted protocol. But there had to be a first time, and that is when I prescribed thyroid medication to a patient who shouldn't have needed it, according to the laboratory. The result must have been successful, otherwise there would not have been a second time. There was a second time and then a third and eventually hundreds and then thousands. What was this successful result? Weight loss. Weight loss that met or at least approached the expectations given the calorie count of the diet. I was comfortable with the consensus of the literature that stated that thyroid hormone would not facilitate weight loss in those with normal thyroid function. The conclusion: Since these supposedly normal patients did finally lose weight, they hadn't had normal thyroid function.

The benefits to the patients didn't end with weight loss. There were other changes in my patients, some of which were as gratifying as the weight loss. I shall presently discuss other benefits of thyroid replacement therapy in hypothyroidism.

I have learned over the years that weight gain often begins with certain events that punctuate our lives, and when that is the case it is more often the result of hypothyroidism than of the irresponsible intake of food. One of the more obvious events is pregnancy. "I never had a weight problem until after I had my first child." One after another, patients have reported this to me. It has become more the rule than the exception.

I have repeatedly probed this circumstance with patients. "Are you sure you didn't eat more after the pregnancy than before?" Generally I hear the same answer. "Is it possible that your physical activity diminished after you had the baby?" "No." I don't mean to imply that this was always the case. Certainly many women have multiple pregnancies and don't succumb to hypothyroidism. But if it is going to occur, it quite often follows the first pregnancy and may indeed grow worse with subsequent pregnancies.

Other events seem to precipitate hypothyroidism. Many patients have reported sudden weight gains after severe emotional shocks or other traumatic events in their lives. I'm convinced that age itself is a factor, though this is a gradual process that takes place over years. Some studies suggest that weight gain accompanying the aging process results from diminished physical activity, but I suspect that there is also a decrease in thyroid function to explain the phenomenon.

Certainly medications play a part. If pregnancy isn't the chief trigger for thyroid-based obesity, then steroids certainly are. By steroids, I'm not referring to the anabolic substances that some weight lifters and athletes are known to use. There are other steroids. They are the cortisone-like substances that are so widely used (probably too widely used) in medicine. These drugs are usually varieties of prednisone or prednisolone and are very useful in treating a host of conditions. Often they are life-saving. Many asthmatics are repeatedly prescribed steroids. Even orthopedic problems are treated with steroids, often by injection into the joints. Of course, this is but another method of introducing them into the body, and although their action is concentrated in the specific injection areas, they eventually enter the general blood circulation.

Because the effect of steroid use is so dramatic, there is a tendency to overuse them when a lesser medication might accomplish the intended purpose. Steroids are drugs that simulate the hormones secreted by the adrenal glands, and their use over time inhibits the normal function of the adrenals. This is a case where the cure can be worse than the disease. At any rate, it is a most common occurrence for me to discover in my hypothyroid patient a history of having taken steroid drugs, often over an extended period of time.

A patient by the name of Jesus provided an interesting variation on the usual case of steroid misuse. He was Hispanic and had been in this country only a few months. His English was probably better than my Spanish, and we did seem to communicate. He should have been losing more weight than he was. He claimed to be doing all the right things. He swore that he stuck to the diet. He was about fifty pounds away from where he should have been and he was losing only three to four pounds a month. There was no question in my mind that he had a very low metabolic rate, and he was already taking a potent dose of thyroid medication to correct it. The dosage seemed right, and he had no signs of overdosage or any other ill effects.

He just wasn't losing. That happens sometimes. There was always the possibility that he wasn't truthful about following the diet or that I didn't understand him fully, but for the most part I rejected those possibilities.

Jesus had a rash on both of his forearms when I first saw him and he told me that he used some sort of cosmetic cream on it to keep his arms from becoming too dry. He was seeing a dermatologist, but he wasn't getting much relief. It looked like psoriasis to me, but I'm not a dermatologist. On his first visit, I had questioned him about any medication he was taking and he said he was taking nothing. As I do with all patients, I had cautioned him that if he were to be prescribed any kind of medication by another doctor, it was imperative that I know about it. I often prescribe appetite suppressants for my patients, and I have to be sure that combinations of medications are compatible.

On one visit, I asked, "How are the arms doing?"

He shook his head. With a grim expression he replied, *"Nada me ayuda,"* which I interpreted to mean "Nothing helps."

(I'm translating.)

"Nothing? What are you doing for it now?" I asked.

"I'm taking these pills he gave me. At first I thought they helped, but I don't think they are working."

"What pills?"

"Those little ones. I have the bottle here."

The medication was methylprednisolone. This is a very widely prescribed steroid prescription with a cortisone-like action. It, like the steroids mentioned earlier, is used for a variety of ailments, everything from joint problems to asthma to allergies. It is frequently prescribed for a six-day period, during which the patient takes six tablets the first day and tapers down daily to one tablet on the sixth day. That's how it had been prescribed for Jesus months ago. The only problem was that Jesus, in order to play it safe, had decided to have the prescription refilled a number of times. He just took one tablet a day after that. I knew that the methylprednisolone was the problem. This wasn't the first time I had seen it interfere with weight loss.

I called for help from one of my bilingual assistants. I admonished Jesus for not keeping me informed of his actions, and he promised to be a good boy in the future. He stopped the methylprednisolone immediately. I explained to him that he should never have continued to take that medication beyond the original prescription period, that it could have other dire side effects beyond the weight problem.

Here is an example of the delicate balance that is maintained by the endocrine glands. The medicine that the other doctor had prescribed and which Jesus unwisely continued to take obviously had an effect on the thyroid. I've seen that same effect with other patients. I've also seen these steroids precipitate weight gain.

Further proof of the negative effect of steroids on weight loss came when Jesus stopped that medication. He began losing at a reasonable rate. The rash would come and go, but he refused to take any more steroids. Eventually he reached his goal.

Another hormone may play a part. Though not as dramatic, it may be that the female hormones that are so commonly prescribed for menopause have a similar effect in lowering metabolism. I'm certain that there is a general relationship between the use of these hormones and weight gain, but I'm undecided as to whether the weight gain is due to hypothyroidism. Perhaps after a few thousand more patients I will have a better idea. Incidentally, birth-control pills are related medications, and the same may hold true for them.

Obesity may not be the most dramatic symptom of hypothyroidism, but it is the one that *this doctor* sees most frequently. I have indicated that I believe about one-fourth of my patients have some degree of hypothyroidism. How does hypothyroidism result in obesity? By lowering your need for calories. If a normal individual needs a certain number of calories per day to maintain weight, then a hypothyroid one of the same stature, age, activity level, etc., needs fewer calories. When one's need for calories is diminished but one's intake of calories isn't proportionately decreased, the result is too many calories and, thus, added stored fat. My patients have all come to me with weight to lose, and quite possibly you're reading this book because of your weight problem. I believe that if you're overweight, there is a one-out-of-four chance that you have some degree of hypothyroidism. As you read on you will learn how to test yourself.

In the process of testing yourself, you may learn that there is no reason for suspicion of hypothyroidism. The test relies upon your body's response to a certain fixed amount of calories. If you respond as a normal person would, we can erase that suspicion and you can get on with the process of losing weight, knowing that it will be no more difficult for you than for any other normal individual.

If the testing indicates that you're somewhat of a borderline case, decisions will have to be made, and those decisions will at least have to be shared with your doctor. Of course he will have to be a cooperative doctor, one who will listen to what you have to say. If the testing leaves little doubt that you have hypothyroidism, then the decision you will have to make is of a different type. You will be faced with getting the right kind of medical help to aid you in losing weight and in reversing some of those annoying symptoms.

Let's not place the cart before the horse. Let's first see how you compare with those who have some of the more common symptoms of hypothyroidism.

Summing Up

- Many overweight people do not overeat.
- Hypothyroidism may be triggered by a variety of factors such as age, pregnancy, or medications.

5

Depression: The Thyroid Connection

I rarely see a patient who has more than a few symptoms of hypothyroidism. I necessarily ignore the patient's weight as an indicator of hypothyroidism, since every one of my patients when first seen is overweight to some degree. Aside from a general "hypothyroid" look, which I've learned to recognize over the years, it is the first few sentences exchanged with a patient that can alert me to the possibility of hypothyroidism.

I will try to describe what I see and feel with this particular type of patient, but the task is difficult and my description may fall short of its mark. For one thing, I expect each of my new patients to be highly motivated at the time of the first visit. After all, my new patient has gone to the trouble of making that appointment and remembering to keep it a week or two later. That morning she groomed herself so as to make the best impression, and she's arrived on time with great expectations that she will once and for all conquer her weight problem. Reconsidering, perhaps she didn't arrive on time. I suspect, but I really haven't kept count, that the hypothyroid patient is more apt to be late than the ordinary patient. That's a sign you won't find in any textbook.

Frankly, I hadn't given much thought to that until I began writing this paragraph.

Perhaps I should comment on why I think punctuality could be significant. Most patients are very excited about starting a weight-loss program. They are enthusiastic. They ask a lot of questions. They want to get it right. They optimistically expect that their lives are about to change. This is the kind of patient you expect to arrive early. Perhaps the best explanation of what I see in the hypothyroid patient is a lack of caring or at least an inability to focus on a task. Being late could be a symptom of that, but I shouldn't read too much into it. After all, the whole thing could also be explained by a traffic jam that morning.

From the onset of our meeting, the patient's lack of focus influences our relationship. Other patients may launch into a diatribe, describing how obesity has interfered with their goals, their discourse often accompanied by expressive body and hand movements. They want to get their message across. They try hard to get me to feel their pain.

Not so with the hypothyroid patient. She is simply there. She states the obvious: that she wants to lose weight. But her declarations lack emotion. It is as though she is lackadaisically reading from a script.

In the course of my patient sessions, I have a number of little "canned speeches" I make. It isn't that I have rehearsed them or that I say the identical words each time, but when you repeat a concept several times each day for years, it does tend to become rather automatic. I generally explain to the patient that weight loss isn't easy. It takes motivation and a systematic adherence to instructions. While I'm reciting this wisdom, the patient will usually make good eye contact and continually nod to show that she is digesting each word. But not the hypothyroid patient. I'm not sure that she is even listening. When I finish a thought, to assure that my message was received I may ask, "Do you understand?" and I will generally get an apathetic nod. In fact apathy might be the best word to describe the aura that surrounds this patient.

The hypothyroid patient's lack of caring sometimes makes me wonder why she is there in the first place. I've concluded that in a very broad sense she does care, but she has trouble sustaining that feeling and expressing the appropriate emotions that should accompany it. She may even have cared more the day she made the appointment and has now forgotten how much she really cared. Forgetfulness seems to be the rule. She generally asks few questions, and when she does, they aren't important questions or useful ones. For example, rather than ask for more specific details on the dietary advice I have given her, my hypothyroid patient may ask, "When do you want me to come back?" or "Can I eat squash?" or other non sequiturs.

A variation on the above is the patient who appears angry or at least annoyed, not with anything specific, but perhaps with life in general. There is a certain degree of good fellowship that usually goes along with a visit to my office. With this patient, it may be absent. My patients aren't acutely "sick." As medical offices go, the atmosphere is rather positive. No one is there to find out if they are afflicted with a life-threatening illness. It is probably as happy an environment as can be expected in a doctor's office, save for perhaps that of an obstetrician. In spite of this, the hypothyroid patient doesn't seem pleased to be there. I wonder if the patient is there reluctantly. Did someone force her to come?

If you think I have chosen extreme examples to make my point, I haven't. Though this emotional affect isn't pronounced in all hypothyroid patients, in some it is even more extreme. It may even have the earmarks of hostility. This is perhaps the depressed patient, who is so well documented in the literature. The mood is also quite changeable; it may sometimes change within the course of one visit. On other visits, there may have been such a difference in personality that I felt like checking the name on the chart to make sure I was seeing the same patient. This could very well be the type of bipolar ailment that is known to be associated with hypothyroidism.

On this latter point, it should be noted that the medication lithium, which is frequently prescribed to treat depressive states and bipolar disease, has been implicated in precipitating hypothyroidism. I've seen a number of patients who had previously been on lithium and who have hypothyroidism. The possibility that there could be a connection is real.

I'm reminded of Mary. My first visit with Mary was pretty much along the lines of the one with the apathetic patient I've just described. She wasn't that much overweight, only about thirty pounds. That's not much in my practice. From the first I didn't have the feeling that we were really communicating. She seemed to be in a fog. A direct question would get a response, but at times it seemed as though she was responding to some other question, one I hadn't asked.

From Mary's routine history form, one that asks a multitude of questions about hereditary factors, past illnesses, habits, medications, etc., I noted that she was taking a mixture of drugs, the ones that are popularly used to treat depression and other psychological problems. In fact, Mary was taking more different mood-altering drugs than I had ever encountered in one patient. She had been seeing a variety of mental-health therapists for years. She described repeated "spells" of depression, during which she "believed" that she ate excessively. She was so vague in her answers I couldn't even be sure of exactly what medications she was taking or who had prescribed each of them. Her current therapist was apparently a nurse practitioner, whom I decided to contact, but I was frustrated in the attempt by Mary's refusal to give me her consent to do so.

I decided to proceed cautiously in treating her. That seemed to be the best course of action, given the whole scenario. For one thing, she was functioning. She did call and make an appointment. She did make it to the office. She did express her purpose in being there, and I thought there was a pretty fair chance that she could follow instructions.

From the first, I suspected hypothyroidism. Not that it was the total cause of Mary's long-standing problem, but perhaps it was a component. During my questioning, she certainly reported many of the signs and symptoms: dry skin, menstrual problems, very thin and dry hair, and she mentioned that she was always cold. When asked if anyone had ever suspected thyroid problems, she answered yes, but everything had turned out to be okay. She couldn't really tell me who tested her or how they did it.

After the examinations, I prescribed an 800-calorie diet for Mary and gave her detailed instructions on implementing it. She wasn't the most attentive listener, but I must say I've seen worse. The first four weeks of treatment of our patients isn't just treatment, it is actually a test of metabolism, and the weight loss achieved during this four-week period is used in calculating the metabolic state. When I saw Mary four weeks later, she had lost only two pounds. I knew from experience that a loss of two pounds meant that she hadn't exactly been faithful to the diet. On an 800-calorie diet, even those with the lowest possible thyroid function lose more than two pounds.

I went through a torturous questioning session that centered around other signs and symptoms of hypothyroidism. Mary had the earmarks, and in fact she was the textbook picture of hypothyroidism. I decided to go out on a limb. I prescribed the smallest dose of thyroid hormone, not so much in expectation of miraculous results, but more as a test of whether it might have any effect at all.

In the first few subsequent visits, I didn't see any improvement. Nor was there any adverse effect. The pulse and blood pressure are pretty fair indicators of negative effects, and both of these were still below what is considered normal. I had gradually been increasing the thyroid dosage during that time. Eventually there was a breakthrough, some weight loss—not much, but it was a hopeful sign. Then on a subsequent visit there was a substantial breakthrough, real weight loss. Accompanying it was an equally impressive change in mood. Over a period of weeks Mary evolved into an entirely different person. She came out of her stupor and gave every appearance of being a normal human being. During that time, on her own, she had stopped taking much of the medication others had prescribed for her.

Eventually, Mary reached her goal weight and was put on our

maintenance plan, which is essentially exercise. The last time I saw her, she said that she didn't have those "spells" anymore, although she did get depressed on occasion. She was continuing with her therapist. I finally spoke to the nurse therapist (with Mary's permission). She was well aware of the changes in her patient. She hadn't realized that the thyroid treatment was in progress. I told her it was imperative that Mary continue taking thyroid hormone. The nurse said she would communicate this to the physician who had prescribed Mary's other medication.

What was accomplished? For one thing, Mary lost her thirty pounds and now feels good about herself, and I'm sure that affects her mood. You don't have to be a psychiatrist to see her psychological improvement. Clearly she has hypothyroidism, and it was exacerbating her psychological problems. She isn't cured, but she is more content, she is responsive, she is definitely functioning better. At least her hypothyroidism is under control.

Mary may be unique, but it is in the sense that every patient is in some way unique. She is representative of the psychological problems that arise from or are intensified by hypothyroidism. I can't tell you how many patients whom I've seen over the years have successfully dealt with their depression through thyroid replacement. I have no way of quantifying my results. I have a gut feeling that many cases of depression that are being treated with the ubiquitous mood-altering drugs are really the result of insufficient thyroid hormone. Even though other drugs may actually combat depression and without a doubt reverse some of the symptoms, their effectiveness may actually be a negative when you consider that they may inhibit patients from attempting to discover the real cause of their problems.

If depression is rampant in our society, so is fatigue. *Fatigue, tiredness, weariness* are words my patients bandy about. They use them to describe the pressures of daily life. That kind of fatigue may show in their faces but not in their step. What they are really complaining of is being overwhelmed, but not actually of fatigue.

Real fatigue is far more dramatic. I can almost differentiate it by watching a patient's gait as she walks into my office. This kind of fatigue is generally present from the moment the patient awakens. Though it may sometimes be delayed a bit, it will generally show up before she is too far into her day. In the last few years, we've been told that there is a new disease that causes fatigue, chronic fatigue syndrome. If it isn't new (it may have been around since prehistoric times), it is now recognized. It has recently been given a name, which makes it easier to talk about.

If you read the medical textbooks on the subject, you will learn that the ailment defies all attempts to find some objective evidence for its existence. The laboratory tests are always normal, or are at least not helpful. If, for example, the hemoglobin concentration is low, then it isn't chronic fatigue syndrome (CFS); it is anemia. If the blood glucose is low, it isn't CFS; it is hypoglycemia. If you run out of tests to perform, it is CFS. What defines CFS is that if the doctor can find no other reason for the fatigue, then it is CFS.

I'm reminded of an exchange that takes place from time to time in my offices. Typically, a patient may tell me that for years she has suffered from a particular complaint and no one knew what was wrong until some very wise doctor recognized it immediately and told her exactly what it was. As an example, let's say the patient has been suffering for years from dizziness. A steady stream of doctors could not find the cause, until finally one guru announced that she had vertigo. Of course, vertigo is simply the medical term for dizziness. Our expert did nothing to help eradicate the symptom, but as long as he named it she thought he was a genius. I have had other patients in whom ringing in the ears was finally diagnosed as tinnitus, whose headaches turned out to be cephalgia, and whose stomach rumbling was eventually discovered to be borborygmus. (Look that one up.) Apparently it isn't very important that you cure an ailment, just as long as you give it an impressive name.

I suspect that many cases of chronic fatigue syndrome are really unrecognized hypothyroidism, unrecognized because the laboratory didn't find it. I have had patients who had been diagnosed with CFS, but the ailment abated after proper thyroid treatment. Is all CFS really hypothyroidism? Undoubtedly not. There may be dozens of other causes. I think we should rename CFS. A more honest name would be "undiagnosed fatigue."

It is estimated that as many as one in ten patients who walk into a doctor's office suffer from depression. Many attempts have been made to define depression and for the most part they are inadequate—the definitions don't encompass each individual case. In essence, depression is vague; it defies definition. Most doctors will admit that there is no hard-and-fast rule for identifying it. Many will admit that diagnosing depression boils down to this: "I don't really know what it is, but I know it when I see it."

It seems that a lot of doctors have seen it and profess to know it. That would account for the enormous number of prescriptions written for such drugs as Prozac,™ Zoloft,™ and Paxil.™ During the taking of the patient's history, a routine question asks what medications the patient is currently taking. It is almost a surprise when the patient replies that she is taking nothing. In female patients (the ones I see most) beyond their teens, possibly half have at some time or another been prescribed mood-altering medications. When asked if the medications had benefited them, a fair number reply in the affirmative, and probably as many others say no.

Though the doctor has prescribed the medication to treat what he sees as depression, the patient sees it as the antidote for stress. Stress is the buzzword generally used to justify why the medication was prescribed. The words *stress, anxiety,* and *depression* are bandied about with little thought as to what they really mean. My patient may be under stress because she couldn't find the right dress for the party this Saturday night, because she didn't get the raise she expected, or because her marriage of twenty-eight years just came to an end. They are all lumped together as the causes of stress. They all result in anxiety. The qualitative and quantitative differences among the causes of stress are ignored. The patient sees the solution to all of these problems as finding the right pill. With the right pill, the dress she wasn't crazy about now becomes acceptable and the husband who had become such a habit no longer seems that indispensable. I have the impression that the physicians' prescribing of these medications is close to a knee-jerk response. The patient utters the word *stress* and the doctor reaches for the prescription pad.

I believe that in many cases there is a relationship between the apathy of persons such as Mary and full-blown depression, in which the individual virtually cannot function. They may both reflect an underlying problem with an underactive thyroid gland. If you will remember that thyroid insufficiency is consistently inconsistent, you will appreciate that a wide variety of moods and psychological problems may properly belong under the same banner. They are either caused by hypothyroidism or they are enhanced by it. I wonder what would happen to the sales of antidepressants if more cases of hypothyroidism were diagnosed and properly treated.

When I prescribe thyroid hormone to my patient because I have determined that her weight loss isn't consistent with her caloric intake, I now have my expectations alerted to more than a weight change. On follow-up visits, I'm more interested in what she has to tell me about how she feels than whether or not she has lost weight. I already know she will lose weight. It is her description of her mood, as well as what I observe of her manner, that tells me that we're on the right track. The weight loss is assumed and is generally there. The bonus is the conversion from apathy to alertness, from a depressed invalid to a functioning human being.

There are those who would argue that the prescribing of mood-altering drugs corrects chemical imbalances in the brain. Likewise, I would argue that when indicated, thyroid hormone corrects the imbalance created by an inadequate amount of thyroid hormone production. Thyroid hormone has a much broader range of activity. Whether its mechanism of action changes the chemistry of the brain is yet to be discovered. It is well known that thyroid hormone treatment is a useful adjunct to other forms of treatment of depression. In my own practice, I've seen it successfully replace other drugs with even more positive results.

In the recent book *The Thyroid Solution* by a well-known endocrinologist, Dr. Ridha Arem, the doctor focuses on how frequently hypothyroidism is ignored as a cause of depression. He takes his colleagues to task for missing the diagnosis. He recognizes many of the reasons for this, some of which I've already alluded to. The laboratory results are given more importance than what the patient has to say. Medical schools have devoted little training to such subjects, and in general doctors are more attuned to recognizing mood problems as psychological rather than hormonal. Dr. Arem makes a strong case for a more vigilant examination for thyroid problems. He and I aren't in agreement when it comes to the value of laboratory testing, and I must stand my ground when it comes to the choice of medications to be used for treatment of hypothyroidism. But Dr. Arem has seen the same shameful disregard of hypothyroidism, and his book could open a lot of eyes.

If doctors would immediately consider the possibility of hypothyroidism when faced with the "depressed" patient, I believe we would see much less reliance on mood-changing drugs and a greater improvement in a broader range of patients' symptoms.

I believe that if more cases of hypothyroidism were recognized and then treated, the incidence of patients under treatment for depression would be greatly reduced. The use of mood-altering medications would consequently decrease, and the only ones who would be unhappy over the change would be the drug companies. As long as we continue to mask one of the frequent symptoms of hypothyroidism with their happy pills, we reduce our chances of diagnosing it.

Summing Up

- Those with hypothyroidism are often listless and apathetic.
- The prescribing of thyroid hormone can often drastically change the personality of those with hypothyroidism.

- Some patients may be assumed to have depression or chronic fatigue syndrome when the problem is actually hypothyroidism.
- Better recognition of hypothyroidism could greatly reduce the reliance on antidepressants in treating depression.

6

Hypothyroidism Woes

Though the thrust of my medical practice is weight loss with perhaps emphasis on those for whom weight loss is problematic because of a thyroid disorder, I cannot ignore the various other aspects of my patients' well-being. I've previously pointed out that those whom I later conclude have hypothyroidism present a wide variety of other symptoms and complaints. I shall discuss briefly some of the more common and troublesome of them.

Infertility

Pregnancy is one of those things that generally brings a weight-loss program to a screeching halt. My practice certainly has its share of pregnancies. Each month my offices can count on a few phone calls from patients who are in the process of losing weight but are now reporting that they are pregnant. They are either congratulated or consoled, as the case may be, but they are always advised to cease our program and to immediately see an obstetrician, who should, for the next few months, be in total charge of what weight-loss regime, if any, is advised.

The subject of pregnancy generally comes up with new patients. I bring it up. I want to be sure our new patient isn't pregnant at that moment. The history I take reviews a patient's past history in terms of how many pregnancies and how many live births she's had, and whether there was anything out of the ordinary with any of them. As you might expect, a certain percentage of these ladies, even though married for a few years, have had no pregnancies. I always inquire as to the reason. Was it voluntary? In a number of cases, I'm told that it was not; in essence, the patient informs me that she is sterile. This leads to a discussion of how she's pursued the problem, and it isn't unusual for the patient to relate the myriad of doctors and tests and even oddball methods that she's been involved in. Generally all this was to no avail.

I usually ask if the investigating doctors considered a thyroid problem. I can generally anticipate the answer. Frequently the reply is that it was suspected (and sometimes, shamefully, not suspected), but that she was tested thoroughly for thyroid problems and when none was found, the doctor went off in other directions. At this point, I don't pursue that train of questioning, mainly because I don't as yet have much of a feel for my new patient's thyroid status. If there are some obvious visible signs of hypothyroidism, I may expound a bit on my opinions of thyroid testing.

Four weeks later, when it is time to evaluate a patient's weight loss as an indicator of the state of her metabolism, I may conclude that this is indeed someone who could benefit from thyroid hormone replacement treatment. It becomes very important that I remember to tell her that although our chief interest is weight loss, she should recognize the possibility that she may become vulnerable to pregnancy once her thyroid problem is under treatment. Patients such as this generally don't use any birth-control methods, either because they would consider a surprise pregnancy a gift from above or because they are so certain pregnancy is impossible that there is no reason to try to prevent it.

Why am I so careful to issue my warning? I haven't always followed that course. In fact, in the early days it didn't really occur to me that there was any reason to warn my patients about pregnancy following thyroid treatment. One surprise after another has made me more cautious. I have had a number of "sterile" patients call me, usually within a month or two of starting on thyroid hormone, to inform me that they were pregnant. Many were delighted. Some were not. Even though some had gone through extensive efforts and expense to get pregnant in the past, they had resigned themselves to the fact it would never occur and had readjusted their goals in life. Pregnancy was no longer part of the plan. Getting pregnant now was a nuisance; in some cases it was viewed as a tragedy. I think some of these people were a little peeved at me. Fortunately, I've never been asked for child support as a consequence of some sort of twisted logic.

Of course now I always warn. And the pregnancies still occur and are generally wanted, but still sometimes they are not. I guess there are those who don't heed warnings. A few years back, Ali was one of the patients I warned.

Ali was a sophisticated European lady of forty-two with a charming accent and matching mannerisms. She was from eastern Europe, where I believe they don't suppress their inner feelings as the British or even Americans are wont to do. A visit with Ali was always a delight.

She had been a patient several years before. She had gotten to a perfect weight and was delighted. There was no effort to restrain herself after that or to follow my advice on how to maintain her figure, and so she returned to my office to start all over again. Ali had no children, had never been pregnant, and had spent a fortune on fertility treatments. For some reason, adoption didn't appeal to her (or perhaps to her husband). This time it appeared that she had developed hypothyroidism. It may actually have been present before, but I was now more accomplished at detecting it. She was put on thyroid replacement with the standard warning: "You might get pregnant." I believe she muttered something like "From your mouth to God's ears."

About six weeks later, Ali announced with considerable fanfare and emotion that her home-pregnancy test pronounced that she was pregnant. I had never seen such elation on my premises. She thanked me up and down and in every other direction. She said she was going to name the child after me. (I felt sorry for any little girl going through life as Sanford.) I advised her that she must see an obstetrician immediately and that she must inform him that she was taking thyroid medication and tell him the dose. I told her that I felt it was necessary for her to continue the medication through her entire pregnancy and undoubtedly afterward. I told her that miscarriages were very common in hypothyroid individuals. I asked her to have her OB call me.

Since Ali was no longer under my care, I lost track of her. She returned about a year later. I realized that she had never informed me of a birth, and I was quite sure she would have let me know. I cautiously asked. She said that two months into the pregnancy, she had had a miscarriage. After that she had been quite depressed. She had gained a lot of weight. Now she was ready to take it off. Her radiant spirit seemed somewhat dulled.

In taking my new history, I asked Ali what her current dosage of thyroid was. She calmly told me that she wasn't taking thyroid. The obstetrician had tested her and taken her off what I had prescribed. She gave no hint that she suspected that stopping the thyroid was a cause of the miscarriage. I certainly suspected it, but I wasn't about to kindle any unpleasant thoughts in her mind. I really think she knew, and I think she knew what I was thinking, but nothing more was said of it. I debated whether to put this incident into this book. I don't think she will mind.

I have other patients who became pregnant while taking thyroid medication under my care. Several have had successfully completed pregnancies, and I believe they had continued taking their thyroid medication.

To sum up, from my experience I believe that hypothyroidism is a frequent cause of infertility. It is often ignored because of reliance on the laboratory to find it. Miscarriage is also the result of insufficient thyroid hormone, and many pregnancies would result in live births if the mother were treated properly.

Not too many obstetricians would disagree with my assessment of the importance of proper thyroid function as a requirement for fertilization and sustaining the pregnancy. Where we obviously differ is in how to diagnose "proper thyroid function" and somewhat in how to treat it.

Of course, infertility in general isn't simply a female problem. A significant number of failed attempts at pregnancy can be blamed on the male, often insufficient production of sperm or other abnormalities of the sperm produced. It would not have been surprising to me if hypothyroidism in the male had been found to result in less or defective sperm production. Yet here again, the thyroid surprises. Studies have shown that hypothyroidism doesn't seem to affect sperm production. Therefore, infertility related to the thyroid gland seems to be strictly a female problem.

Menstrual Problems

Even more frequent than infertility in hypothyroid patients are menstrual problems. If you recall, I have told you that the inconsistency of the symptoms of hypothyroidism is the only consistent characteristic of the ailment. You would expect menstrual abnormalities to accompany any affliction that resulted in infertility, and you would be correct. The menstrual abnormalities that accompany hypothyroidism run the whole gamut of such problems.

While one hypothyroid patient will complain of the complete absence of periods for long stretches, perhaps years, another will report two or three periods per month, and not with any regularity. The complaint may be of a very heavy flow, or it could just as frequently be of a scant flow. In many cases that time of month becomes a major traumatic event because of the discomfort. Far beyond what is described for premenstrual syndrome, the patient could become completely nonfunctional. She misses work, cannot concentrate, and is impossible to live with.

Some women seem more willing to accept what they regard as a curse than are others. Some relentlessly pursue one effort after another to get to the bottom of their trouble. I think this is more apt to occur when pain is the major component. That isn't surprising. Some of my patients have had every test imaginable. X rays and MRIs are commonplace. Virtually everyone in this intense category has had all the thyroid tests. A number have had D & Cs, a sort of last-ditch effort on the part of the gynecologist. I even recall that some patients have gone through exploratory abdominal surgery to find the cause of their painful periods, but with no positive finding or result.

Do you encounter the phrase "I know it when I see it" as frequently as I do? It seems as though it's being used more and more. It expresses one's frustration with not being able to define clearly something that should not be very difficult to define. For example, the head of Personnel might say, "I don't know how to describe the characteristics of a good employee, but I know it when I see it." That's the way I feel about many patients with hypothyroidism. My description of them feels inadequate, yet I know it when I see it.

I should explain that I don't *always* know it when I see it. Often I'm fooled. That's one of the characteristics of hypothyroidism, and that's consistent with its inconsistency. Still, if I had to guess, I would say that in five minutes with a patient I could guess right about 60 to 70 percent of the time. If I were to make a guess in those five minutes and my answer were to be yes, it would be much more reliable than a "no" answer. That's another way of saying that in a number of cases the manifestations of the problem are very atypical. I'm fooled a lot when the patient doesn't display any outward signs. The one defining characteristic, the slow burning of calories, is the one that isn't obvious in those five minutes.

I guessed no for Monise. I would have expected her chart to say, under Occupation, movie star or model, or perhaps former model. Instead it said medical assistant. Yet, she was overweight, though only by thirty-five pounds for her five-foot-five-inch height. Don't be troubled by my use of *only*. I do that a lot. That's how I see 5'5" and 162.

Monise was full of life, as bouncy as they come. No hypothyroidism here, I thought. I was wrong. She seemed to have it all except for two things. One was her weight; the other I was to learn later. The first month her weight loss was a dismal three pounds. Monise swore she had deviated only once from that 800-calorie diet during the whole month, and that deviation was a single slice of pizza. Her three-pound weight loss told the story. It was inadequate. Later, I will show you how I knew she had a thyroid problem from that little bit of information. That is an important element in the test you will be doing on yourself.

I had generally somewhat ignored the part of her history where Monise noted that she had painful periods. After all, I'm not a gynecologist and she didn't come to me for that. I didn't completely ignore it, but I must have reasoned that it had other causes. This lady's manner and appearance were very uncharacteristic of the more typical hypothyroid patient. When I saw her at that first four-week visit and encountered the three-pound loss, I became more interested in her periods. She told me that the whole experience was frightful. She had such pain that she was obliged to miss work at least two days a month. The doctor she worked for, a gynecologist, said that this happens in some women, and he had put her on birth-control pills. It helped only a little, but that was when the weight gain started. She blamed the pills for the weight problem and that is why she stopped them on her own. She obviously chose the pain over gaining weight. She elaborated on one additional point of interest: She was always cold.

It was clear enough that for this lady, three pounds in four weeks spelled hypothyroidism. Her menstrual problems and feeling cold were confirming evidence. I prescribed thyroid hormone. Four weeks later, there was an eight-pound weight loss; that was adequate. She was ecstatic, as I expected, but not about that. She reported that she had had her first pain-free period in years. No pain. To her it was a miracle. I had previously told her that there was the possibility that the prescription might help her periods, but I don't think she took it seriously. The rest of the story was uneventful. She got down to her goal weight, 127. Her periods were no longer a problem, and my guess is that she has maintained her weight. I know that her gynecologist continued to prescribe the thyroid hormone I had started her on.

There was a lesson in this for me. It reinforced what I had known for a long time. There is a delicate balance when it comes to trusting your own intuition in these matters. More specifically, go along with that gut feeling when you think the patient is hypothyroid, and don't trust it when you don't think so. You might very well be surprised. Yet, looking at the broader picture, I don't really need to rely completely on my intuition; the test I developed does a lot of the work for me. Still, it's a nice feeling when you guess right and really help someone.

When it comes to reversing the symptoms with proper treatment, there is a high degree of success when the cause is hypothyroidism. It is almost routine for a patient to tell me how improved that last period was. She will volunteer this information even though she didn't feel inclined to complain about the problem previously. I've seen every one of the manifestations of these previous paragraphs reversed by the prescribing of thyroid hormone. Particularly gratifying is that the patient doesn't have to wait very long to see the result. In some cases, the reports of improvement are actually seen during the first month.

Interestingly enough, I've seen patients who have come to me already on thyroid therapy but who still had menstrual complaints. In the course of my treatment, if I found it necessary to increase the dose of thyroid in order to facilitate a more normal rate of weight loss, the patient would often report a concurrent improvement in her menstrual difficulties. Improvement seems to be dose-related. When the patient gets the right amount of thyroid, the problems improve.

Coldness

Are you always cold? Of course no one is *always* cold, but do you complain frequently of being cold? Do you get into arguments with family members or fellow workers about turning up the heat or turning off the air conditioning?

If you or someone else meets the above description, it would be a bit premature to declare hypothyroidism immediately, but I'll bet you will be right more often than wrong. The fact is that hypothyroid people are apt to complain of being cold. I've never seen a reasonable explanation in the scientific literature for that symptom, although it is certainly well recognized. If I had to come up with an explanation, I would say that it isn't surprising, since it is like many other body parameters in hypothyroidism. Low rather than high seems to be the rule in hypothyroidism.

Remember, my belief is that the common denominator of hypothyroidism is the inability to burn calories at the "normal" rate. Since the thyroid gland controls the rate at which metabolic processes proceed, it would seem logical that if less fuel were consumed, less heat would be generated. The hypothyroid individual doesn't just feel cold, *he or she is cold.* We've already learned that. The body temperature is often reduced a degree or more in hypothyroidism. That was even the basis of Dr. Broda Barnes's test for hypothyroidism.

This reduction in metabolic processes can be seen in other areas. I expect my hypothyroid patient to have low blood pressure, and more of them do than don't. This is in spite of the fact that an overweight individual generally is more inclined to have an elevated blood pressure. Thus, when an obese patient has a low blood pressure, it is a double surprise. Normal blood pressure would have been unexpected, but low points the finger at the thyroid.

The rate at which the heart beats in the hypothyroid patient is just one more clue, if not a confirming finding. As you may know, a slow pulse often heralds someone in fine physical condition, quite often an athlete. Activities that make our pulses race barely change theirs. My overweight patient is out of shape and has to strain just to do ordinary tasks. A fast pulse would be usual during every activity, with the possible exception of sleep. Yet I'm apt to see just the opposite. Here is someone who outweighs me by a hundred pounds, doesn't do a lick of exercise, and her pulse rate is slower than mine. On the surface, that seems like an injustice, but it isn't. She is still paying the price for her weight, it is just not obvious from the usual vital signs.

The only vital sign that doesn't seem to be reduced in a hypothyroid patient is the respiratory rate. At rest, we're supposed to breathe in the neighborhood of sixteen times a minute. Inevitably, my patient has a rate of twenty or more, and when physically stressed, she will puff at an impressive rate.

I have spoken of the generally relaxed appearance (I restrain myself from calling it a stupor) of the hypothyroid patient. Every motion is slow, not so much deliberate but rather like watching a motion-picture film that is slowed just a little. Muscle movement generates heat. Since our hypothyroid individual moves minimally, less heat is produced. The counterpart is the athlete. A runner must dissipate the heat his effort produces by transferring it to the air that surrounds his body. We have a very efficient cooling system that depends upon the evaporation of our perspiration into the air to keep us at a cozy temperature. Depending upon weather conditions, the runner's body may not be able to rid itself of that heat, and during his run he may have quite an elevated body temperature.

Feeling cold and being cold are just part of the generalized underfunctioning of the hypothyroid individual. When the problem is reversed, generally by addition of thyroid hormone, the body temperature rises, the complaints of coldness become fewer, and all the other processes increase or speed up. Coldness is thus not so much a symptom as a manifestation of the combined effect of a group of other symptoms.

Fibromyalgia, or "I hurt everywhere"

Fibromyalgia is believed to be almost as prevalent as I believe hypothyroidism to be, and I suspect that it isn't a coincidence. That's a lot of people to suffer from a disease that wasn't even recognized as a disease fifteen years ago. If you search medical textbooks written before that time, you will find nary a word about fibromyalgia.

Pain, stiffness, and muscle fatigue are the earmarks of this widespread problem. Specialists who deal with muscles and bones and joints and nerves have been deluged with such complaints for years, but since, as in the case of chronic fatigue syndrome, with which it is often associated, there was little that the laboratory could do to pin down an ailment, it was very slow to be recognized as a disease. Of course the ailment has probably been around for centuries, but, as with hypothyroidism itself, the signs and symptoms were so many and varied that it overlapped a host of other conditions. In short, we didn't have a name for it. The literature certainly describes similar conditions and calls them such things as fibrositis or myofascial pain syndrome. Years ago, one doctor developed a unique method of treatment that involved injecting anesthetic agents into very small painful areas, which she called trigger points. This technique has gained a reasonable amount of popularity and does seem to provide relief.

The pain is in the fibrous tissues of the body—muscles, tendons, ligaments, fascia—which is another way of saying it can be anywhere. In some it seems to locate in several "favorite" spots, while in others it acts capriciously. One minute pain is here and the next minute it has moved elsewhere.

Eventually the American College of Rheumatology recognized fibromyalgia as a specific disease entity and set forth criteria for diagnosing it. A major element in this diagnosis was the physician's ability to elicit pain by applying pressure to the numerous particular trigger points, specific sites known commonly to be associated with the reported pain of fibromyalgia.

It has been noted that fibromyalgia is found very frequently in those with hypothyroidism. Of course, every time I read a paper or book that makes reference to that fact, I must bear in mind that the author is probably defining hypothyroidism by the most widespread method, and that is the interpretation of laboratory reports. At least one author differentiates between fibromyalgia in those *with* hypothyroidism and in those *without*. I make the presumption that he, like many others, is referring to hypothyroidism as confirmed by the usual laboratory tests. Since I've rejected that method as the single positive means of labeling a patient as hypothyroid, I'm not sure I'm ready to accept the distinction between those who have or don't have hypothyroidism. I believe that if all fibromyalgia isn't the result of low thyroid function, then at least a much greater percentage of it than is generally accepted does result from an absence of thyroid hormone.

I shall not go into the woes of fibromyalgia beyond saying that it is a hodgepodge of pain that can be anywhere or everywhere, pain that changes location at the drop of a hat and defies all efforts to eradicate it. The literature describes a collection of symptoms that turns out to look a lot like the corresponding list for hypothyroidism: headache, constipation, painful menstrual periods, depression, etc. Fibromyalgia is said to be frequently associated with chronic fatigue syndrome, and this isn't surprising since constant pain would certainly result in fatigue, whether physical or mental. Everyday painkillers can help and antidepressant medication is often used to treat it, but that is hardly a cure. If anything, by lessening the symptoms, physicians thwart any effort to investigate the cause earnestly.

I don't diagnose fibromyalgia in my patients. My prime purpose is to take weight off of them. Many come to me and report that fibromyalgia has been diagnosed by another doctor. Almost without exception, they haven't been treated with thyroid hormone because it was ascertained that they weren't candidates for it. Some of them are eventually put on thyroid by me in response to their demonstrating an inadequate response to the diet they've been following. I've never prescribed thyroid hormone to treat fibromyalgia per se. Yet I've seen many favorable results in terms of these complaints of pain in those in whom it has been diagnosed. Strangely, these particular patients aren't overly demonstrative over the flight of their pain; they simply take it in stride. I think many of them attribute the improvement to the weight loss and not to correcting the thyroid problem. That's all right. I'm certainly not sure what caused the change, but this improvement in aches and pains definitely seems to occur in my hypothyroid patients.

One chiropractor seems to have made a strong case for hypothyroidism as the cause of fibromyalgia. He advocates prescribing T3, one of the thyroid hormones. Another M.D. thyroid specialist reports that he has had very good results with a combination of two hormones, T3 and T4. Later, I will be discussing these medications, as well as one other.

I would like to see someone study the effects of thyroid hormone in patients who show *symptoms* of fibromyalgia and *symptoms* of hypothyroidism but who have gotten a thumbs-down from the laboratory on the latter diagnosis. I think there is an opportunity there for some researcher to really make a name for himself.

The connection between hypothyroidism and fibromyalgia and the fact that there is such an overlap of signs and symptoms seems to me beyond coincidence. That effective treatment of the former seems to also have a positive effect on the latter is something we cannot ignore.

And More

I believe we don't suspect that many other patient complaints are really manifestations of hypothyroidism. We know that anemia, headaches, constipation, impotence, and even brittle fingernails can also be a part of it. Skin and hair problems are also frequent.

The skin of those with hypothyroidism has a certain puffiness to it. It looks like it is loaded with water, and it probably is. Dryness is a regular complaint, yet I've seen cases where the skin was oily. When I see hair that seems lifeless and possibly unmanageable, I take note. That reminds me of Helen.

The first time I saw Helen I was impressed by several things. Her weight alone didn't impress me. I've already seen too many five-foot-four ladies who weigh in the neighborhood of 243 pounds. What first caught my attention was how well groomed she was. It is often difficult for people that heavy to do a satisfactory job of looking nice. For one thing, the right clothes are hard to find. It strikes me as unusual that in a society with so much obesity, a lot of marketers don't take advantage of this. In general, clothes seem to be designed for thin people. Helen was one of the most handsomely groomed new patients I had ever met.

Another thing that was different about her was that she carried an attaché case. At the risk of sounding like a male chauvinist, which I'm not, the plain fact is that most women that come into my office carry a handbag. She didn't, only an attaché case. Soon, that was easily explained. She was an attorney. She presented a very professional image; her grooming, her attaché, her posture, the assurance in her walk, all contributed to the image of someone who is important. By the time I had seen Helen several times, I couldn't help noticing that her hair was particularly well coiffed. It was always perfect and the hairstyles seemed to vary a lot. She also changed hair coloring during those first few months. I guessed that she invested a lot of her earnings in the hairstylist.

She told a less than remarkable life story. She had been on every diet imaginable and had made the rounds of the weight-loss establishments and the diet doctors. A few years back, a doctor had said he thought she needed thyroid hormone, and he prescribed it. She didn't think it helped much with the weight loss and so eventually she didn't renew the prescription. Later, more than one doctor said that there was no thyroid problem.

There was. I prescribed thyroid medication again, but this time natural thyroid rather than the synthetic hormone she had taken years before. She didn't have many other symptoms of hypothyroidism. The fatigue she complained about could just as well have been caused by carting all that weight around. She did complain of falling asleep at the drop of a hat, a circumstance that had more than once proved inconvenient in the courtroom.

Helen needed the thyroid treatment and she was reasonably well motivated. In the months that followed, she lost weight nicely and seemed to be happy with her progress. I complimented her on that progress regularly. Sometimes I would also compliment her on her hairdo, and she accepted that graciously but without any desire to dwell on the subject.

Her thyroid dose had to be adjusted upward in a couple of steps, and we settled on a satisfactory dosage. It was the better part of a year before she told me her deep dark secret: *That wasn't her hair.*

I really don't know if the women on my staff knew this; women have a way of discerning such things. I certainly didn't. I was shocked when she told me, but I've learned to maintain my composure when a patient shocks me. That isn't an infrequent event.

"Why didn't you tell me earlier?"

"I don't know. I was embarrassed."

"Is there a problem with your own hair?"

"There sure is. I don't have any. Correction, I didn't have any."

"What do you mean?"

"For years I had a hair problem. It was so thin that there were big bald patches. I couldn't go out in public that way. I have the biggest collection of wigs you've ever seen."

Then it came out. Helen's hair had been growing back. She said it was almost presentable. She would not let me see it. I had to take her word for it. She knew immediately that the thyroid hormone was responsible for the new hair. She was knowledgeable. When I first told her she had hypothyroidism, she read up on it. She had been optimistic that her weight would benefit from the treatment, but it was too much to hope that her hair would as well. To say the least, she was delighted, but in a dignified way. She had a very professional manner about her and she wasn't about to jump up and down.

A few months later, I got to see Helen's real hair. Shortly after I walked into the treatment room, I made one of my usual comments about her nice hairdo. It came out with one of those knowing glances we display when we know we're sharing a secret.

"You're wearing your hair shorter these days."

"You noticed."

"Of course. It looks very nice."

"It is my hair."

"What?"

"*It is my hair.* My real hair."

We shared warm smiles.

I've tried to give you an overview of hypothyroidism and its manifestations. As if we don't have enough already, I've no doubt that between the time I write the last word of this book and the time it reaches the bookshelves a few more signs and symptoms will be added. Hypothyroidism is indeed the Greater Imitator.

I haven't dwelled on any of these other signs and symptoms because my chief interest is how it affects your weight. From here on I will concentrate on that aspect of hypothyroidism.

Summing Up

- Infertility is often caused by hypothyroidism.
- In the course of treating hypothyroidism, "infertile" women may become pregnant.
- Menstrual problems may be completely reversed in the hypothyroid patient who is treated properly.
- Feeling cold could be a sign of hypothyroidism.
- Multiple aches and pains often diagnosed as fibromyalgia may be eliminated by the use of thyroid hormone.
- A variety of other conditions, such as skin and hair problems, often respond well to thyroid treatment.

7

Natural or Synthetic Treatment?

In an earlier chapter I told you that the cause of hypothyroidism is that the body receives an insufficient supply of thyroid hormones for it to function properly. For our purposes, it isn't fruitful to argue whether the thyroid gland isn't doing its job or whether the problem is on the receiving end, that is to say, whether the various sites where the hormones act respond to the quantity of hormones available. The effect is the same: The body needs more thyroid hormone. It has been shown repeatedly that when the supply of thyroid hormone increases, the signs and symptoms of hypothyroidism are eradicated or at least improved.

The process by which we supply the body with hormones from external sources is popularly referred to as *hormone replacement therapy.* Every female who has entered menopause or who is close to that time has undoubtedly been exposed to the debate regarding whether estrogen replacement therapy is advisable. And it *is* a debate. Some doctors lean one way, and others in the opposite direction. There isn't too much argument as to whether supplying estrogen and sometimes other female hormones improves the annoying baggage that goes with menopause. It is more a question of whether supplementing the patient's hormone production from the outside is risky. The patient's history as well as her family history often play an important part in the doctor's decision.

When a diabetic injects the hormone *insulin,* it supplements the patient's own inadequate production of the hormone and allows the patient to function. Indeed, it may be life-saving. That is another type of hormone replacement therapy. The supplementation of a patient's own supply of thyroid hormone from a source outside one's own body is perhaps not quite so dramatic, but tell that to the sufferer of hypothyroidism. The changes that ensue can indeed be remarkable.

Nothing is more exciting to me than medical breakthroughs—medical firsts. I suppose there is a first time for anything. We recognize that the ability to create fire was one of the great milestones in the history of the human race. There must have been a first time when a human being intentionally did what was necessary to produce the spark he captured in some twigs that resulted eventually in a fire of his own making. It's a shame we don't know who he was so his name could have been enshrined in the books. I wonder if he had a name!

There was a first time a human being was supplied with thyroid hormone from an outside source. Before I tell you how and when it came about, I should first tell you why it was done. The recognition signs of hypothyroidism have been noted for perhaps a thousand years. We may not have had a clue as to what caused that excess weight or those abnormal menstrual periods or that overwhelming fatigue, but we knew that these symptoms, along with others, were sometimes present in combination in certain people, and that they did constitute some discrete unknown ailment. For most of the nineteenth century, the condition was referred to as myxoedema (sometimes the "o" is omitted). We still speak of myxedema today, but generally differentiate it from hypothyroidism as a more severe form of the latter. Much of the scientific literature that I've researched from the late 1800s and early 1900s lumps all hypothyroidism together as myxoedema.

In 1891 a doctor by the name of George R. Murray was the

first to inject a thyroid substance from an animal (a sheep) into a human patient. The lady suffered from myxoedema with more of the classic signs of the ailment than are generally present, among them lethargy, slow speech, menstrual problems, and sensitivity to cold—in short, the works.

The improvement could not have been more dramatic, and so was born the modern treatment of hypothyroidism. True, we no longer strain the stuff through our handkerchiefs, but the treatment today is essentially what Dr. Murray started. What had been born was thyroid replacement therapy. Murray's success fostered a flurry of activity among doctors, and the following year no less than three doctors, working independently, showed that you could achieve the same effect by giving the thyroid juice by mouth. Since then we've certainly refined the product and its method of manufacture, and there has been some variation in the composition of the hormones used, but surprisingly little.

Preparations containing thyroid hormone slowly became available to the practicing physician. They underwent some name changes. At the turn of the century *iodothyrin* from sheep was what doctors were using to treat hypothyroidism. Pharmacology books of the era readily admitted that its actual constituents were essentially unknown. By 1915, *Glandulae Thyroideae Siccae, U.S.P.* was an established product. The "U.S.P." stands for United States Pharmacopeia, a prestigious designation that establishes standards for the quality of medications. What eventually emerged in this country was Thyroid U.S.P., a standardized material that was extracted from the thyroid glands of animals we use for food: sheep, cows, and hogs.

Thyroid U.S.P. has been available for many years in tablet form, and it comes in a variety of strengths. This allows the physician a lot of versatility when prescribing thyroid. I began prescribing Thyroid U.S.P. to appropriate patients back in 1957 when I first began my practice. It was always gratifying to see a patient respond to proper treatment, and nothing made more of an impression on me than the response to thyroid treatment in a patient who really needed it.

There are other names for natural thyroid. It is often called desiccated thyroid. (Desiccated means dried.) Very often it is referred to as Armour Thyroid or simply Armour. This comes from its history. For years it was supplied by the Armour meatpacking people. Today it is manufactured by Forest Pharmaceuticals. Unquestionably, Armour is the most well-known name for natural thyroid.

There weren't many choices when it came to treating an underactive thyroid. The thyroid hormone I was prescribing for my patients wasn't much different from what Dr. Murray injected into Mrs. S. I'm sure mine was cleaner and I had a better idea of how much thyroid hormone was in each pill. Of course, he didn't know there was such a thing as thyroid hormone, but his thyroid juice accomplished the same purpose. I liked using natural thyroid on my patients, but I did have another choice.

During my first year in practice, synthetic thyroid hormone became available. There is an ongoing disagreement among our population as to the merits of "natural" as opposed to "synthetic" substances. Everyone from food producers to cosmetics hucksters proudly flaunts the word *natural*. *Synthetic* has virtually acquired the synonym *unnatural*. Should we take natural or synthetic vitamins? Do we really like synthetic fabrics? Some do. Ask any sky diver what kind of parachute he prefers. Natural doesn't always win out. There is certainly a common bias when it comes to natural versus synthetic, for example, with fur coats. Yet, overall, natural seems to win the popularity contest.

Synthetic thyroid received more attention than would have been expected. There was a good reason—or at least a reason that explained this, good or bad. As effective as treatment with natural thyroid had been over the years, there was periodic grumbling about it. There were many reports, perhaps justified, that the physician could not rely upon the strength of the tablets. The actual potency didn't always seem to correspond to the strength printed on the label. In most cases, it was believed that the therapeutic effect was less rather than more than what was expected. There were reports that patients might be doing well with a prescription, but with refills they would find that the medication didn't seem to work as well. The doctor might then increase the dosage, perhaps by telling the patient to take an extra pill, and the situation would improve. Perhaps with the next refilling, the new dosage would appear too strong, the patient would have symptoms of being overmedicated, and the dosage would then have to be reduced. I'm reporting what was the prevalent thinking of many medical men. My own experience with natural thyroid was quite different.

An explanation for this mistrust of natural thyroid seemed to make the rounds. The problem was staleness. It was said that thyroid medication would deteriorate in potency as it sat on the pharmacy shelves. If you had your prescription refilled, you wouldn't know whether the product you were getting was fresh and potent or whether some of its potency had been lost. A major selling point of the synthetic preparation was that it was very stable and maintained its potency throughout its shelf life. Each year, its use increased, at the expense of natural thyroid. This confidence in the standardized nature of synthetic thyroid has lasted even to the present day, even though many physicians are unaware that the confidence they have in it should have been seriously shaken by what occurred just a few short years ago.

The "synthetic" thyroid hormone I have been speaking of is actually levothyroxine, or, more properly, levothyroxine sodium, which is commonly designated as T4. One manufacturer of this product dominates the market and receives most of the cash spent on thyroid medication. This is the product that boasted stability, reliable potency, and safety. In 1997, the government exploded the myth with this statement published in the *Federal Register:*

> . . . [N]o currently marketed orally administered levothyroxine sodium product has been shown to demonstrate consistent potency and stability and, thus, no currently marketed orally administered levothyroxine sodium product is generally recognized as safe and effective.

What followed was a flurry of legal activity in which manufacturers of levothyroxine sodium were required to clean up their acts. Since overpayment for the products was an issue, class-action lawsuits were filed against manufacturers, and eventually there was a $41.8 million settlement.

I must say that I had never experienced any variability of thyroid medication with my patients. I was aware that there had been such a complaint against natural thyroid, and since I was seeing a sizable number of hypothyroid patients even after one year in practice, I decided to guard against "drugstore staleness" by obtaining my thyroid medication directly from the manufacturers and dispensing to my patients myself. In that way I knew that what I was dispensing was fresh. I didn't know whether the anecdotes about thyroid pills were true, but I decided to play it safe.

My natural curiosity finally got the best of me. I decided to begin prescribing synthetic thyroid to some of my patients. Everyone else was doing it. It seemed that I was out of step with progress. Those to whom I gave synthetic thyroid actually belonged to two groups. There were patients who clearly had hypothyroidism whom I had been treating for some time. Some of these had been diagnosed by a previous doctor and I was continuing their treatment with the synthetic thyroid he had prescribed. If I had to adjust the dosage up or down, I would do so.

Then there were some patients whom I arbitrarily switched from natural thyroid to synthetic. In making such a change, there is an entirely different dosage to be reckoned with. The manufacturers of the synthetic product publish what they believe to be the comparable dosage, so the job is somewhat easier.

Almost from the first, I suspected that I wasn't giving my patients the comparable dosage. The error was virtually always in one direction: The patient didn't seem to be getting enough of the hormone. That seemed easy to correct. I increased the dosage of the synthetic product. Yet even in doing so, I didn't get the same effect. The patient would voice her dissatisfaction, saying that she was becoming more fatigued, much as she had been before thyroid treatment. Perhaps her periods had become irregular, as before, or they were prolonged, or particularly painful. Some patients were very insistent that I switch them back to natural thyroid. Some were even angry that I had chosen to rock the boat.

There were occasions when I increased the dosage and the patient would then report symptoms that suggested I was giving too high a dose. A well-known sign of overdosage of thyroid hormone is a tremor of the hands. About the only time I have ever seen this was in some of the patients whose dose of synthetic thyroid hormone I was trying to adjust.

Another group to whom I prescribed synthetic thyroid were patients who had previously undiscovered hypothyroidism. Prescribing synthetic thyroid from scratch was much the same experience as it was in the other group. I had become accustomed to what to expect in the way of improvement with thyroid therapy, but it wasn't the same with these patients. Synthetic thyroid didn't seem to work as well as I had come to expect. It wasn't particularly as a result of my own observations that I came to this conclusion, but rather as a result of reports from the patients themselves.

I have never since gone back to prescribing synthetic thyroid from scratch, but I've continued to prescribe it to patients who had received it from other doctors. Over the years, many new patients of mine had been taking synthetic thyroid at the time of their first visit. I'm always reluctant to fix something that isn't broken, so if they have no complaint and seem to be doing well, I leave things as they are. If, however, it appears that they aren't getting sufficient thyroid, I will generally supplement the synthetic thyroid they are taking with my prescription for additional natural thyroid. They are thus taking a mixture of the synthetic and the natural. Often this works out quite well. If I'm still not satisfied, I may discontinue the synthetic and replace it entirely with what I believe to be the equivalent dose of natural thyroid.

I don't mean to suggest that synthetic thyroid doesn't work. It could hardly have achieved such widespread acceptance if it were of no value. But my own experience is that it doesn't work as well overall. If this is a personal bias, it is an honest one. Many of the improvements we see in a patient's condition are quite subjective, on the part of both the doctor and the patient. My hypothyroid patients feel that natural thyroid consistently works better, and I must trust their observations.

The names given to the various thyroid medications can be confusing. The following box may help.

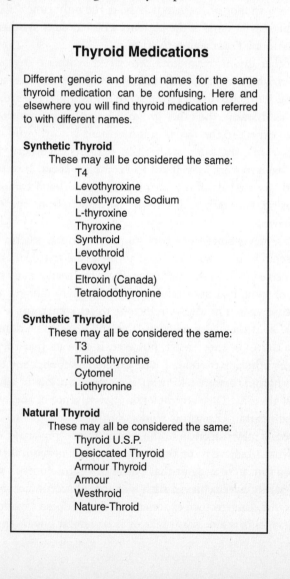

Thyroid Medications

Different generic and brand names for the same thyroid medication can be confusing. Here and elsewhere you will find thyroid medication referred to with different names.

Synthetic Thyroid
    These may all be considered the same:
        T4
        Levothyroxine
        Levothyroxine Sodium
        L-thyroxine
        Thyroxine
        Synthroid
        Levothroid
        Levoxyl
        Eltroxin (Canada)
        Tetraiodothyronine

Synthetic Thyroid
    These may all be considered the same:
        T3
        Triiodothyronine
        Cytomel
        Liothyronine

Natural Thyroid
    These may all be considered the same:
        Thyroid U.S.P.
        Desiccated Thyroid
        Armour Thyroid
        Armour
        Westhroid
        Nature-Throid

I'm reminded of one experience involving natural thyroid. The patient's name was Gladys. It isn't that her case was much different from hundreds I had seen before and since, but I remember her very well. It is strange how you can forget a patient you saw last month, but others stay with you permanently.

Here was someone sincerely wanting to lose weight. She was sixty-five pounds over her acceptable weight. She was a systems analyst, a very responsible job dealing with computers. Her first visit wasn't the typical apathetic request for help in losing weight. She was agitated. She recounted how it just didn't come off. She had been to every diet facility imaginable. Nothing worked.

I'm wary of a patient who presents this type of history. This is the kind of person I'm ready to label as having psychological problems. She sees things very negatively: every treatment is either inadequate, or improper, or too expensive, in short—a rip-off. It may be administered by incompetents, or the facility is too inaccessible. She will always find some deficiency on which to focus. Having such excuses essentially gets the individual off the hook. After all, it isn't her fault she didn't lose weight. It was the fault of those programs she tried.

At first glance, I could have written her off as belonging to that not uncommon group. Not so. There was a difference with Gladys. She had given each of her treatment providers an adequate chance. She didn't stop because of the usual reasons. She stopped because she wasn't losing weight. She stopped treatment in each case when it became apparent that nothing would be accomplished by continuing the program. In fact, it was sometimes the program that gave up on her.

Gladys was quite pretty. She was neat in appearance and she must have given much thought to her wardrobe. You would not suspect that she had sixty-five pounds to lose. I knew from her history that she was single. She didn't talk about her social life or her sex life, as many patients do. I don't bring up the subject. I wait for the patient to do that. She was quite likable. I imagined that she had a social life.

I recall that Gladys had been to several doctors. She had been tested repeatedly. She was told her thyroid was normal. This is akin to saying she just ate too much. She knew she didn't. I don't recall that any of the physicians came right out and accused her of lying, but she felt the inference was there. She came to me on the recommendation of a friend who had been successful at losing weight with me. She was probably not hopeful that anything different would happen under my care. It is just that she wasn't yet ready to throw in the towel.

I sound sympathetic and I truly was. My relating to her that I had little respect for thyroid testing was sort of a shot in the arm. That got her interested. She believed she had a thyroid problem, and she came right out and asked me if I would give her thyroid hormone. She was very knowledgeable when it came to thyroid. She had done some reading. Of course, she also knew that the TSH test was considered the benchmark of thyroid diagnosis, and she had had a lot of normal TSH results in her life. As I recall, one of the previous tests indicated an overactive thyroid, one that is more likely to render the victim thin.

She appeared hopeful that I might treat her for hypothyroidism, and she was visibly disappointed when I told her it wasn't that simple. I had to have better evidence that her thyroid function was low. The first month of treatment was to be the test. She agreed, but her spirits were somewhat dampened by the delay in attacking the problem head-on.

I had the feeling from the beginning that I could rely on what this lady had to tell me. I was impressed with her sincerity coupled with her intelligence. She wasn't the typical apathetic hypothyroid patient. In my own mind, this lessened the odds that we would find hypothyroidism, but I kept an open mind, knowing the inconsistent nature of the illness.

Gladys's weight loss at the four-week visit was a meager two pounds. She recited the same earnest oaths of conforming 100 percent that I've heard so frequently. I believed her. She had eaten 800 calories for twenty-eight straight days and had lost only two pounds. That translated into a maintenance level of calories of 1,050 a day—remarkably low.

She knew the significance of all this and didn't waste any time in asking me, "Will you give me thyroid now?" This time the answer was yes. But I didn't acquiesce before questioning her several more times as to how she might have deviated from the diet. She stuck to her story. She had eaten 800 calories a day for twenty-eight days.

Gladys was started on one-half grain of natural thyroid per day. When she saw the medication that had been prescribed, she called me. She politely was questioning what I had given her. She knew what thyroid hormone looked like. She had seen pictures of the pills in books and had even known others who were taking it. She knew that the various doses of thyroid were of different pastel colors. The tablets I had prescribed were a dull, off-white shade. She wanted an explanation. I gave it to her.

What she was familiar with was synthetic thyroid, the commonly prescribed tablet, also known as levothyroxine or just T4. I told her that I had prescribed for her natural thyroid. She hadn't heard of that. I had to go into an explanation of how I felt that it was a better medication than the synthetic. I'm not sure she bought it. I think she was losing confidence. She agreed to follow through.

I had one more phone call during that next week. She had been doing some homework. She had read in some article that natural thyroid was an old drug that wasn't used much anymore because the synthetic variety was better. This didn't sit well with her. Why was I giving her inferior medicine? I had to explain that in my opinion, what I had prescribed was superior to the other. She of course was relying on the printed word. It is impressive how powerful is the printed word. It didn't matter that I had umpteen years of experience. When someone writes something and it gets published, it becomes truth. I was a little disappointed in Gladys. I thought she was smarter than that.

But the situation changed dramatically on her next four-week visit with me. She had lost five pounds. I wasn't delighted, although I thought we were making progress. She, on the other hand, was overjoyed. She seemed to think that was the most she had ever lost in a like period of time. The task of dealing with her intensity now became much easier. I upped her dosage to one grain a day. There was no evidence of any ill effects from the medication. The only other sign that we were getting somewhere was her report that she no longer seemed to need a sweater at work. Everyone else had been comfortable, but she had always been cold. She hadn't told me about this at the first visit. It certainly could be a significant finding.

It is terribly trite to say that the rest is history, but I will say it anyway. In the months that followed, Gladys's weight loss was consistently over ten pounds per four-week period. She reached her goal weight rather painlessly. She was the talk of her office. Incidentally, I hadn't realized what her potential was. I think she could have qualified as a supermodel. To my knowledge that wasn't her desire. I remember speaking to her family doctor at the time I discharged her. It was an uphill battle getting him to continue the thyroid I had prescribed. I must have been pleading. When he learned I had prescribed natural thyroid, it didn't make the job any easier. I doubt he had ever written a prescription for natural thyroid, but I prudently didn't ask him. He could not deny that the story I had told him was persuasive. He finally agreed, but said he would proceed very cautiously. That was a bigger triumph than getting her straightened out. I wouldn't be surprised if he eventually switched her to synthetic thyroid, but that's all right. Gladys will probably do fine with that.

Gladys wasn't that unusual a case. If anything was different about her case, it was that the problem was solved quite easily. I had determined that she had very low metabolic activity and I was expecting that the dose of thyroid would have to be increased considerably before any real results could be obtained. The first increase in dosage was all that was needed. It strengthened my suspicion that there is somewhat of a threshold dosage that works for each hypothyroid individual. Until you reach that dosage, results are inconclusive. Once you cross the threshold, magic happens. This is my hypothesis; it's unproven, but this seems to be the case.

Another nice thing about treating Gladys was that she was so compliant that it established the validity of the treatment so decisively. Had she been a troublesome patient or lacked motivation, there would have had to be a lot more heart-to-heart discussions. Here was a lady who knew what she wanted and went right to the task of accomplishing it. I wish all my patients were like Gladys.

Why has the pendulum swung so strongly in favor of synthetic thyroid? I truly don't know the answer. I can only guess. I know that marketing must have played a part. I know that in speaking to various doctors over the years, I've been surprised at how many shared my opinion of the superiority of the natural product. What is more puzzling is the fact that in spite of this, they were still more apt to prescribe the synthetic. I suppose there is a tendency to find safety in numbers. I suppose most doctors aren't comfortable with prescribing what the majority of their colleagues are not. Remember, in terms of official recognition, Thyroid U.S.P. is still, as ever, a reputable product. It is simply not prescribed that much.

There is another possible explanation for this apparent paradox. Perhaps it is best explained by quoting from Goodman and Gillman's textbook on pharmacology from 1965. I might point out that this textbook was the standard for pharmacological information at the time. Keep in mind that synthetic thyroid hormone had been available and in wide use for about seven years. Here is the book's assessment of a reason for the prejudice directed at natural thyroid:

> Thyroid U.S.P. is a highly satisfactory preparation for clinical use. Its continued popularity doesn't derive merely from a reactionary attitude, although at first sight the preparation might seem to be crude, old-fashioned, and poorly standardized. It is evidently uniformly well

absorbed unless it has an enteric coating, and the potency is sufficiently standard that variation cannot be detected clinically if the official preparation is prescribed. A few years ago a large batch of material came into the hands of a number of distributors in the United States and Europe and, although of proper iodine content, it later proved not to be thyroid at all. The episode gave thyroid a bad name because several publications about the unreliability of thyroid were made before the hoax was uncovered. Recent analyses indicate that the triiodothyronine in thyroid contributes significantly to the thyromimetic effect, and this may in part explain the greater effectiveness of the product than anticipated from its content of thyroxine.

Several things are notable about this passage. Notice that it talks about the "greater effectiveness" of this product over synthetic thyroid (thyroxine or T4), which by then was in wide use. That is totally consistent with my own observations. Has something changed since 1965? If natural thyroid worked better during that era, could it be less effective today? Both products are still the same as they were then.

The above quote does point out how rumor and innuendo play such a role in forming our opinions and our biases. Natural thyroid may never have recovered from the adverse publicity. I wonder how many physicians who have graduated from medical school since, let us say, 1965 have ever prescribed natural thyroid or have had any personal experience with it. In fact, I wonder how many are even sure it still exists and is available to them.

In my own practice, natural thyroid, or Thyroid U.S.P. as it is properly called, is the medication I use to treat hypothyroidism. I believe doctors should take a new look at thyroid replacement therapy, consider whether they are getting the optimum results from their patients with their current course of treatment, and, above all, try this long-standing and still approved medication on some of their patients.

I'm going to go into a perhaps more persuasive reason why natural thyroid deserves serious consideration. In the quotation above, Goodman and Gillman suggest that the triiodothyronine in Thyroid U.S.P. significantly contributes to its effectiveness. I've spoken to you of triiodothyronine earlier. For simplicity we call it T3. The other major thyroid hormone found in your own thyroid gland as well as in natural thyroid is T4. Synthetic thyroid contains only T4. Let's be sure you understand the lineup. Natural thyroid contains both T3 and T4, while synthetic contains only T4. The Goodman and Gillman textbook suggests that natural thyroid is superior because of the additional T3. Dr. Siegal concurs, but he isn't the only one.

In the first piece of scientific literature in a long time to substantiate my position, a paper published in the February 1999 *New England Journal of Medicine* indicated that T4 alone didn't work as well in the treatment of depression caused by hypothyroidism as the mixture of T4 and T3. Although the researchers didn't specifically advocate the use of natural thyroid to supply the two hormones, they did report the benefits of the mixture. They apparently used the two hormones as individual substances in combination. This is but a short step away from using natural thyroid, which normally combines the two.

This paper has great significance. First because it was published in our most prestigious medical journal, a publication known to accept only the highest-quality work. Second, it seems to confirm what many of us have had faith in. You may expect much follow-up and fallout from that article.

Actually the follow-up began within the same issue of the journal. The study was commented on in an editorial, which took the position that the study was promising but conservatively concluded that we should not switch our patients to the combination of two hormones yet. The editorial author seems to have ignored the fact that the "switch" was made years ago. Using one hormone, T4, was a switch away from using the two hormones. Remember that both hormones are present in natural thyroid, which was the acceptable standard for years. More correctly, the editorial writer could have advised, "Let's not go *back* to two hormones yet." He seems to believe that the ratio of T4 to T3 should be about 10 to 1, but he doesn't explain how he came to this conclusion. In the study he is commenting on, the ratios of T4 to T3 given to subjects varied considerably. Strangely enough, the ratio of T4 to T3 from thyroid hormone derived from cows has been shown to be a little over 9 to 1, very close to what he feels is ideal.

Perhaps an even more important substantiation of the value of natural thyroid comes from what I believe to be the most important of the sources: the patients. I've told you that when my own patients have had the opportunity to compare the effects of natural and synthetic thyroid they overwhelmingly choose the natural. This preference doesn't come from my patients alone. There are a number of Web sites where extensive information about thyroid problems is available. Here, organizations dealing with thyroid problems disseminate information, but there are also a number of sites that are essentially conducted by laypersons. One of the best is apparently the labor of love run totally by Mary Shomon. Among her many offerings is the exchange of information and comments from viewers who suffer from thyroid problems. It is my observation that the majority of her viewers seem to have hypothyroidism. You only have to monitor this site for a few sessions to realize the general discontent of many of them toward their physicians. It is surprising how many of these people are quite knowledgeable when it comes to natural thyroid.

One of the offerings on Ms. Shomon's Web site is a letter written by a patient, Shirley Grose, to her doctor. She had no compliments for him. He apparently made disparaging statements about the Armour Thyroid she had been taking. He refused to prescribe it for her. The lady had done her homework. In her letter to him, she may have made a better case for natural thyroid than I have. She demanded answers as to how he substantiated his opinion of her natural thyroid preparation. I wonder if she ever received those answers.

I have had a number of patients who would have liked to have sent similar letters to their former doctors, but they may not have had the research or writing skills of Ms. Grose. As a result, they vented their feelings on me. I think they would have applauded her saying to her doctor, "I would like to know why you thought I was unqualified to say how my own body felt."

A fuller version of Shirley Grose's story is found in Appendix J.

On that same Web site, viewers actually seek help from others in searching for doctors who will prescribe natural thyroid. Sometimes they make reference to a "Barnes" type of doctor.

I have mentioned Dr. Broda Barnes previously. He's probably been the most critical of some of the dogma surrounding the recognition and treating of hypothyroidism. In his 1976 book, *Hypothyroidism,* he chastises the doctors who rely on the laboratory tests in preference to responding to the obvious symptoms of the patient. Clearly, Barnes used natural thyroid to treat his patients. He gives dosages only for natural thyroid. Yet nowhere in his book does he actually compare natural with synthetic thyroid. He virtually ignores the existence of synthetic thyroid. I cannot help but speculate as to this omission. It isn't logical that a doctor writing about hypothyroidism would not even mention the then most common drug used to treat the ailment. It smacks of an intentional omission. Was some sort of pressure exerted upon him to ignore the medication he didn't endorse? Was this a politically correct position forced upon him? A few years back, I made an effort to locate him and ask him the question. I was too late. He had passed on.

Though Dr. Barnes is gone, the Broda O. Barnes, M.D., Research Foundation, Inc., is dedicated to carrying on his work. In their literature they seem to affirm that he was critical not only of blood testing for thyroid problems. According to them, his position on medication was:

> Patients taking thyroid replacement therapy have much better improvement to symptoms with natural desiccated thyroid hormone rather than synthetic thyroid hormones.

Here's a story that seems apropos. I've treated a lot of husband-and-wife teams over the years. This generally works out very well. They tend to keep each other motivated. Sometimes I suspect that competition spurs each of them on. They generally, but not always, support the efforts of their mate. If the husband is about to throw in the towel, the wife will often give him a pep talk and get him on the right track.

A man might come to me after his spouse has already been a patient. The wife might come home and say, "Honey, it's about time you lost weight too. It's terribly bad for your health. I want you to make an appointment with Dr. Siegal." That rarely works. He'll make the appointment all right to satisfy his wife, but the motivation isn't there. This is the type of case that generally doesn't end in success.

Some pairs are wonderful. I'm thinking of Sherwin, Fran, and Armando. That's not a pair, that's a threesome. Armando is the fifteen-year-old son. Fran came first. This fifty-three-year-old lady had only twenty-five pounds to lose. At the end of two weeks, the scale showed she was down nine pounds, a clear signal that there was no thyroid problem. Her husband and son made appointments. When teenagers make appointments I always speak to the parents first. Below age fifteen, I tend to discourage the parents from pursuing the medical route. From experience I have learned that at that age there is very little motivation do what is unpleasant. It takes a certain level of maturity to have the discipline necessary to diet. Kids just don't have it. And I don't want them to fail. I don't think that failure at that age is healthy. (Is it at any age?)

Nonetheless, I accepted Armando as a patient. He seemed more mature, more adult, than many of my adult patients. It turned out that he was just that. He took the no-nonsense approach to dieting and in three months lost forty-two pounds and was put on a maintenance program that was essentially a lot of exercise. Patients like Armando make it all worthwhile.

I didn't learn that Sherwin was himself a physician until I saw him for the first time. I have to confess that I find physician-patients generally trying. I'm always sure they are suspiciously evaluating my every move, just as I do when I go to a physician. As much as I hate the idea, I suspect I'm not myself at these times, and this embarrasses me. Sherwin gave me no reason to feel self-conscious. He acted like any other patient. If I hadn't been told he was a doctor, I wouldn't have known.

Worse than that, Sherwin was a specialist in internal medicine. I must tell you how unusual that is. He was the first—not the first physician I'd treated, but the first internist. I've had scads of doctors as patients and they've come from a variety of specialties. I don't know why internists don't darken my door, but I imagine they have no reason to think I know more about losing weight than they do. (All this is just speculation.)

Dr. Sherwin weighed 248 pounds and he was five feet nine inches tall, with a medium build. A proper weight for him would have been about 160. He was by far the most serious case of the three. His first month's weight loss was only six pounds. He said he'd been totally compliant, and that meant he was a candidate for treatment with thyroid hormone. I expected opposition to the idea. He had had our usual battery of lab tests, but they didn't include thyroid tests. I awaited, "What, no thyroid tests?" But he didn't say that and there was no opposition. I kept thinking, Why is he not asking me the obvious? I prescribed his medication. He didn't act differently than any other patient in these circumstances. To boot, I had prescribed natural thyroid. I was willing to bet he had never written a prescription in his life for natural thyroid. But I'm sure he had written a million of them for synthetic thyroid.

Sherwin had to have his thyroid dose adjusted a couple of times, and eventually the weight came off quite well. After the first forty pounds he mentioned that he hadn't known that it was possible to feel so well. He has referred many patients to me. The whole family was a success story, and yet as I look back, I can't help but wonder. All the internists I know diagnose hypothyroidism by the book. They don't prescribe natural thyroid. I would like to have known why he was so accepting of treatment that I knew he didn't give to his own patients. I wanted so to know, but I never had the courage to ask. (If he reads this, maybe I'll get my answer.) I wanted to know why Sherwin never questioned my methods. I've treated many other doctors and we always get into "doctor talk." I remember asking my receptionist after his first visit, "Are you sure he's a doctor?"

When Sherwin was discharged, I mentioned that he would have to continue taking the thyroid medication. He asked me for the exact information as to dosage and said he would obtain it himself. And that was that.

Sherwin will always be a mystery to me, but a pleasant one.

I believe that natural thyroid will again regain its popularity. I don't see how the good results I have been getting from it for so many years can be ignored. A combination of new research, patients' feedback, doctors willing to listen as well as others willing to speak out, can make the change.

In a later chapter as well as in the chapter for doctors, I will explain how I use natural thyroid to treat hypothyroidism.

Summing Up

- Natural thyroid hormone has been in use for over 100 years for treating hypothyroidism.
- The synthetic hormone, though effective, is not as effective as the natural hormone.
- There has been an unwarranted bias against natural thyroid.
- Many hypothyroid patients are aware of the difference between the two and request natural thyroid from their doctors.
- Most doctors are unfamiliar with natural thyroid and choose to prescribe the synthetic variety.

8

The Usual Way and the Better Way

If you've ever made a visit to a doctor, and who hasn't, you've probably at one time or another had some laboratory tests performed. To learn more about you, it is certainly standard procedure for your doctor to go beyond what he can see, feel, or hear. That's where laboratory tests come in.

When we think of laboratory tests, we tend to think of blood tests, where someone inserts a needle into a vein and withdraws some blood, which then is subjected to strange and mysterious analysis. There are other procedures that still fall under the realm of lab tests, and these have nothing to do with blood. Still other lab tests involve the examination of other body fluids. There are also tests that have nothing to do with removing any body fluids or other pieces of you. Your eye doctor might do various tests that could probably be classified as lab tests in which he may not even make physical contact with you. A stress test is one where your heart's response to physical exertion is monitored. Since we're presently interested in your thyroid gland, you should know that all tests relating to the thyroid aren't simply blood tests.

We, of course, are concentrating on a particular aspect of your thyroid gland. We would like to know whether it is supplying you with enough of its thyroid hormones. The words in the last sentence were chosen precisely. Your thyroid gland may indeed be supplying a "normal" amount of the thyroid hormones, but we're interested in knowing whether that amount is "enough" for you.

Remember, two thyroid hormones are known to regulate our metabolism. We've called them T3 and T4 for short. T3 is much more potent than T4, but it is present in the thyroid gland in a much lesser amount. It acts very quickly upon the cells that receive it, and then it dissipates rapidly. Because of this fast action, the patient gets somewhat of a jolt after taking it and in a sense becomes *hyperthyroid* for the moment. This can produce undesirable side effects. T4, on the other hand, is slower to act and is converted inside the cells to T3 before it performs its regulatory functions. Because of this more gradual action, most doctors prescribe T4 alone to treat hypothyroidism, the disease characterized by an inadequate supply of the hormones.

It is only logical that we would like to know just how much T3 and T4 are in a patient's bloodstream. Logic tells us that if the amounts are lower than normal, that should certainly account for hypothyroidism. The situation becomes more complicated when you realize that there is another endocrine gland involved in all of this. The pituitary gland, often referred to as the master gland because it exerts much regulatory effect upon the whole endocrine system, produces a hormone called thyroid stimulating hormone, a name generally shortened to TSH. It is believed that the pituitary gland monitors the amount of T3 and T4 in the circulation constantly, and when it finds that the amount is "subnormal," it releases its hormone, TSH, into the bloodstream. The name given to TSH suggests what happens next. The thyroid gland, in turn, monitors the amount of TSH in the bloodstream, and when that amount increases, it is stimulated to release more of its hormones into the bloodstream.

A perpetual cycle is thus created. When the pituitary senses that there is an abundance of T3 and T4 in the bloodstream, it stops releasing TSH, and when the thyroid senses this drop in

TSH, it stops releasing T3 and T4. This reciprocal process is what is believed to regulate our metabolism.

Since two glands are involved in this process, it should be clear that a problem with either of them could upset the balance of this delicate regulatory mechanism. By assessing the amounts of the three substances involved, T3, T4, and TSH, doctors hope to figure out what the problem is and where the problem is. That all seems quite straightforward, and it would seem that it isn't that difficult to analyze one's thyroid status.

Let's look at some theoretical laboratory results and then think through the meaning. For simplicity we will look only at a couple of combinations of T4 values and TSH values. Suppose the amount of TSH in the blood is determined to be higher than normal, and at the same time the amount of T4 is lower than normal. We could conclude that the low T4 meant the thyroid gland wasn't putting out enough T4. The high TSH value tells us that the pituitary gland is aware of this and is trying to get the thyroid gland to increase its production, but obviously that isn't happening. That should tell us that the problem is with the thyroid gland and not with the pituitary. The pituitary is doing its job, but the thyroid gland is not. That's clear enough, isn't it?

Suppose both values are low, the TSH as well as the T4. It looks like the thyroid gland isn't putting out enough T4, but since the pituitary isn't putting out TSH in order to stimulate T4 production, suspicion falls on a defective pituitary. Of course, both glands could be malfunctioning, but that is less likely.

Most doctors have great confidence in the conclusions that they draw from such lab results relating to the thyroid, and this seems very clear-cut. If it looks like the patient isn't getting enough thyroid hormone, supply it to her. I've lost track of how many tests of thyroid function I have done over the years. Even though I've done tons of them, you've already been told I have little confidence in them. Why? As I've just explained, the theory seems sound. But things don't always work as they are supposed to work.

For one thing, some of the tests of thyroid function are known to be unreliable if the patient is already taking thyroid medication, and the fact is that many of them are. They may be told that they must discontinue taking the medication for varying periods of time in order to get accurate results, and the literature certainly differs in what those time periods are. The thyroid hormones are carried in the blood combined with a protein called thyroid binding globulin. If there is too much of this substance or perhaps not enough of it in the blood, it definitely can affect the lab findings for T3 and T4. Doctors often have to test for thyroid binding globulin in order to reinterpret the T3 and T4 results.

Of course, another possibility for error is the same possibility that exists for all lab work, namely human error. I have, for example, sent blood specimens from the same patient drawn on successive days and gotten such varied results that no conclusions could be drawn. There is an even more curious phenomenon that occurred on several occasions. On these occasions, determined to get to the bottom of my displeasure with the lab results I was getting, I decided to take the blood specimen from a particular patient and divide it into two different portions, sending them both to the lab, but under different fictitious names. The reports always gave somewhat different results, sometimes with very large discrepancies.

The real problem may be quite remote from any of this. Is the amount of thyroid hormone circulating in the blood really all that important? It is recognized that the hormone does its work only when it reaches the cells that will be affected by it. Is it possible that cells in one person react differently from those in another? Could there be a defect not in the thyroid or its hormones, but in other parts of the body so that they don't take proper advantage of the hormone? I don't know the answer. Certainly that explanation has been suggested.

It became apparent to me that given the doubts I had about the reliability of the lab, I needed to look in other directions if I were to be able to help these overweight patients who also had many of the signs and symptoms of hypothyroidism.

I have said that blood tests aren't the only kinds of laboratory tests. When I was first in practice, a very well accepted test of metabolism and presumably thyroid function was the BMR test, which stood for basal metabolic rate. The word *basal* referred to a baseline, the patient's condition when she was at her most serene and relaxed. It was generally assumed that this was when the patient awoke in the morning, before eating anything, and before encountering the stresses of the day.

We would see the patient as early as possible, before breakfast, ask her to lie on a treatment table in a darkened room for a half hour or so, and we would then quietly and calmly hook her up to an apparatus. It had an oxygen mask. There were varieties of these machines that doctors used to run this test. I remember that one of my machines had a sort of clothespin gadget we used to squeeze the nostrils shut so that all breathing, in and out, was through a tube placed in the mouth. The machine measured the amount of oxygen the patient consumed over a period of time and also measured the amount of carbon dioxide she expelled through the mouth. From these figures a calculation was made, and we could tell the patient something like this:

"Your BMR result is minus-twenty-three. This means that your metabolism is low. You're what is called underactive. We need to start thyroid treatment."

That's all there was to it. The test was very popular. It was being done left and right. Eventually it began to lose favor. The theory itself was sound enough, but the problem was the technique of administering it. It was supposed to measure the patient under basal conditions. This hardly meant after she had gotten up, made the bed, showered, brushed her teeth, done her hair, made breakfast, gotten the kids off to school, and then had driven ten miles in traffic to the doctor's office. The half hour or so of rest in the office was supposed to nullify those stimulating effects. It was argued that the only way to do the test properly was for the doctor to be at the patient's home when she awoke, and then immediately attach the mask and begin. Obviously, this wasn't too practical. I'm not sure that if one of my patients awakened to find me glaring down at her it wouldn't influence the result, or, worse, precipitate a heart attack.

No one argued that the best place to do the test was in the hospital, where the patient had stayed overnight. This was frequently done. Of course, that ran up the cost. Certainly much of the criticism of the test was valid; I never did have a lot of confidence in the results. Still, I acted on the results if my own observation of the patient was consistent with the BMR result. Again, the theory was sound enough but the implementation was difficult.

I'm not sure that the theory behind blood tests is quite as sound. On balance, as flawed as the BMR was, I think I had more confidence in it than I have in blood testing. In spite of the fact that the most authoritative textbook on the thyroid of the 1970s devoted twenty-three pages to that test alone, by the end of that decade the BMR test was fading into oblivion.

It was replaced by something rather bizarre. Did a doctor ever hit you with a little chrome hammer that had a triangular red rubber head? Aside from allowing him an outlet for aggression, this test does have some useful purpose. Certain reflexes are diminished and sometimes accentuated with various ailments. The doctor might tap your leg just below the knee and you would both watch that involuntary kick. There is a similar reflex that we all have that involves the tendon that runs up the back of your leg from your heel. It is known that in hypothyroidism there is a delay in the relaxation phase in this type of reflex after the hammer taps that tendon. Opportunistic people invented machines to measure this time delay. The patient was asked to kneel on a stool while the tester used one of those hammers to tap the Achilles tendon. The foot would jerk and the machine would take its measurement of one phase of that movement of the ankle. I have to say that I found this very useful. I think the results were quite valid. They seemed to coincide with my own observations of the patient. For some reason or other, the whole method fell out of favor; my machines eventually needed repairs and there were no longer parts for them, nor was there anyone who knew anything about them. So much for Achilles reflex testing.

There is another kind of testing that is quite different from any I've described so far. I particularly like this kind of test because it deals with what the doctor sees, feels, and hears while he is with the patient. In 1969 a group of researchers from Scotland wrote a paper in which they reported on how they had used their own senses (really only three) to diagnose hypothyroidism. The test is usually referred to as the Billewicz index, although six others co-authored the paper. The test was based solely on observation of the patient. It included the patient's history as well as what was observable. They listed thirteen signs of symptoms of hypothyroidism (mental lethargy, dry skin, constipation—you should know them by now). They then listed eight physical signs (dry skin, slowing of ankle jerk, etc.). They then evaluated each patient for each of these signs and symptoms. They very cleverly gave more weight (importance) to some than to others. The result they called their diagnostic index.

No blood tests, no expensive machines, just observations and common sense. Of course nothing is without its problems. The researchers used a control group, which is another way of saying that they wanted to compare the scores of those whom they were testing and whom they knew to be hypothyroid with the scores of the control group, whom they knew didn't have hypothyroidism. The problem, as I see it, is that they determined who had it and who didn't have it in advance by using the results of the then accepted blood tests. Ironically, years later there are papers published that use the Billewicz index as a check of the validity of blood-test analysis. Think about it. Isn't there some sort of endless-loop nonsense afoot?

Yet I like the Billewicz approach. In fact, I like it so much that I've included a concept derived from theirs in Chapter 13, "Evaluating Your Metabolism." The difference is that there is no preconceived impression of whether you have the problem or not. We start from scratch. You take the test, then we decide whether you have the problem.

I have spoken of Dr. Broda Barnes, the doctor who wrote a book all about hypothyroidism and who some might believe wrote it entirely with a poison pen. He was terribly critical of his profession when it came to thyroid. At any rate, Dr. Barnes had his favorite test. He knew that those with hypothyroidism have a low body temperature. So he took his patients' temperatures. That doesn't seem all that inventive, does it? Actually, he didn't do it himself. He had them take their own temperatures. He placed great value in this. Dr. Barnes's patients' body temperatures were a major consideration when it came to diagnosing them. I've said that I thought this method had merit. Perhaps I'm not quite as enthusiastic as Dr. Barnes about it, but it does make sense. You will hear more about this later.

Is blood testing useless? I guess I'm not ready to say that yet. Certainly many patients are tested by conventional means, put on therapy, and many of them do quite well. My complaint is that many cases are missed or ignored because of the blood-test results. If I won't admit that blood testing is useless, do I feel it is useful? In my experience, not very. I think there are better ways. I think the Billewicz test has value. I think Dr. Barnes's temperature test is useful. In combination, the individual value of each test is probably multiplied. I also think that the test I use on my patients, the one that gets right to the heart of the matter, is the most valuable. You will be able to decide for yourself.

I will describe briefly the Metabolic Function Index test, but there is much more about it later in the book. If you decide to take the test, you will be asked to eat a diet of 1,000 calories per day for a four-week period. You will lose weight on that diet, guaranteed. The question is, how much. Based on how much you lose, with some simple arithmetic, I will show you how to calculate how many calories it takes for you to maintain your weight, that is, not to lose or gain. You will then compare that amount with how many calories it *should have* taken you to maintain your weight. There is little math involved in all this. It's not very difficult. Your sixth-grader should be able to do it.

Your Metabolic Function Index, your MFI, will be expressed as a percentage of normal. If you turn out to have an MFI of 100 percent, you don't have a metabolic problem. If it turns out to be 75 percent, you do have a problem.

The reason I have so much confidence in my test is that it goes right to the crux of the problem. There is nothing hidden. It is really quite simple. Here is how it works: If it is known that hypothyroid individuals don't burn sufficient calories, let's eat a certain number of calories and then let's see how fast we burn them up. That's all there is to it.

In Chapter 11 you will get the exact details of how to run this test on yourself.

Summing Up

- Over the years, there have been a variety of tests to determine the state of one's thyroid function.
- Not all thyroid tests have been blood tests.
- The metabolic function test in this book investigates the problem directly by comparing one's own burning of calories with that of a "normal" person.

9
Why Protein for Weight Loss

You cannot help but have noticed that there is a lot more being said about protein diets than there has been for many years. In fact, if you're a sufficiently young adult, you may not be aware that high-protein diets were once very popular. Is it not evident that there are varied opinions on what role protein should play in our diets?

During my growing-up years, I think there was every bit as much interest in diets and getting thin as there is today. But there was a difference: People weren't as intense when it came to searching for the "magic" cure for obesity. Sure, there was plenty of nonsense around, even then. One of my hobbies is to collect memorabilia of weight-loss schemes that were popular through the years—you know, articles, advertisements from newspapers or magazines, that kind of thing. Even a hundred years ago you could buy soap that would wash out your excess fat. There were batteries, magnets, and even the makings of tapeworms could be purchased in capsule form. But the purveyors of all this stuff weren't nearly as sophisticated as our current crop of vendors.

One of the reasons most of the newspaper and magazine ads for weight-loss potions and devices didn't seem to attract a sizable audience was that everyone knew how to lose weight without this outside help. There was no mystery. Maybe folks were no more apt to follow what they believed to be the proper weight-loss diet than they are today, but there was little doubt among the masses as to how to lose weight. As a result, even though there were a few diet books around, their approach was the usual conservative advice on sensible eating, and they really didn't sell very well.

Of course, diet books have been around for a long time. Even though there is dietary advice widely dispersed through the Bible and it is present in other ancient writings, the first real diet book came from England. In 1727, Dr. Thomas Short wrote a treatise titled *Discourse Concerning the Causes and Effects of Corpulency.* It's fun to read. Among other things, he believed that bad air was partially responsible for "corpulency" and advised his readers not to live near marshes. The first diet book that had any kind of readership also came from England, but 136 years later. William Banting had battled obesity for years. He was disappointed in the medical attempts to cure him until one doctor apparently gave him the right diet. He was so impressed with his results that he rejoiced by printing a pamphlet, his *Letter on Corpulence,* in 1863. It told the world about the diet that finally worked for him. For a frame of reference of the times, our Civil War was going on then. Americans were too occupied, but the English took his advice to heart. At least at first, he distributed it free. Perhaps because the price was right, the pamphlet was a "best-seller."

Banting's *Letter* had such an impact that it was the standard of diet in England as well as the United States for perhaps fifty years. The medical men didn't particularly like it, but eminent physicians debated its value in the most prestigious journals for half a century on both sides of the Atlantic.

The Banting diet wouldn't excite anyone today. For one thing, it is quite vague. Dr. Banting virtually didn't specify quantities for many of the foods he recommended. There was no doubt that it was a high-protein diet. Banting had his readers eating lots of meat, fish, and fowl. About the only things he excluded from those categories were pork and salmon. He recognized that they were quite fatty. Banting's diet was rather low in carbohydrate. He forbade things in that category: bread, sugar, potatoes, and beer. He did allow two or three glasses of wine, a concession that may have contributed to his popularity.

I have said that during my formative years everyone knew how to lose weight. What I mean is that they knew the general principles, and I believe that those principles owed much to Banting. What they knew was that the best diet food was protein: meat, fish, and fowl. We also knew what made us fat. Strangely enough, it wasn't fat. I think everyone knew that fat carried a lot of calories, but the real enemy was an abundance of carbohydrate. We knew that if you wanted to get thin, you had to curtail the bread and potatoes.

A milestone in promoting this concept was the Holiday Diet of 1950. It wasn't a diet to follow while on vacation. It got its name from *Holiday Magazine,* then the top travel magazine. A Dr. Pennington who worked for the Du Pont company apparently had great success with reducing overweight employees there. He was written up in *Holiday,* and there were even follow-up articles. The magazine was deluged with information about the diet. What was the diet? You can sum it up in one word: meat. The dieter was to eat a half pound of fat meat three times a day with minimal accompanying vegetables. If the meat wasn't fat enough for his liking, Pennington advised how to add more fat to it.

Pennington wasn't unique. Before and after, others were advocating similar diets. Dr. Blake Donaldson, in a charming book called *Strong Medicine,* informed us that

> there are only two absolutely necessary foods for humans—fresh fat meat and water.

Restaurants at the time didn't ignore the needs of the overweight client. Diet plates were very common. What would you expect to find on them? A meat patty and perhaps a green vegetable or a salad.

I started practicing general medicine in 1957, and I couldn't ignore the prevalence of obesity in my practice. By 1960, I had all I could do just to handle those who were overweight, so I decided to limit myself to just that type of patient. In 1968, the first very big diet book in ages came out. It was written by a really cute old doctor by the name of Irwin Stillman. Cute? Sure. He was a frequent visitor on the late-night talk shows. Everyone loved him because he said funny things. His diet? You guessed it: lots of protein and virtually no carbohydrate. That, at least, was Dr. Stillman's basic diet. The problem is that he had so many alternate diets in his book that I don't see how anyone could have made a decision as to which one to follow.

What I've been trying to get across is that for an important segment of our history, high protein and low carbohydrates were the standard methods of weight loss. This wasn't limited to the public's perception of what to eat to lose weight. The majority of doctors subscribed to the same concept. If there was any controversy, it had to do with fat. Some said eat it; others said don't.

In the 1970s things began to change. Meat fell into disfavor. We started hearing more and more about complex carbohydrates. Self-styled gurus (in a sense we're all self-styled) started singing the praises of low-protein, high-carbohydrate, and low-fat diets. Protein was tolerated in limited quantities, but fat was the real enemy. Exercise was promoted and the gyms proliferated and prosper to this day, although membership certainly dwarfs participants. Little books that told you how much fat was in each morsel of foods you might eat were for sale at all the checkout counters. In previous decades, similar books told you how much carbohydrate was in your foods so you could reject those that had more than a smidgen. Now we were being told to load up on carbohydrates.

What resulted? It is obvious from the patients I see. My impression: *We as a society have never been fatter than we are today.* If the carbohydrate craze wasn't the cause, it certainly wasn't the cure. One after another, my patients were telling me they had tried this diet and that diet and the only thing that happened is that they got fatter and fatter. Strangely enough, they didn't seem to blame the diet. Instead, they believed there was something wrong with their bodies. After all, they had followed the advice that had been given them. They were too young to know that this kind of advice changes from decade to decade, and even if they did know it, they believed that the most recent advice was always better than all that old stuff.

Among the experts, there is a lot of support for the proposition that a calorie is a calorie and it doesn't matter if it comes from an animal or a plant or lettuce or butter. There has been a mountain of research done during the first half of the twentieth century concerning whether carbohydrates, proteins, and fats were indeed interchangeable in the diet when it came to supplying energy (calories). No one disputes how much energy (how many calories) the individual food groups contain. We know that carbohydrate and protein each store 4 calories per gram and that fat stores 9 calories per gram. (There are about 454 grams in a pound.) The question arises that when we eat each of these, do we end up with those amounts? The most dedicated and thorough research was done years ago to answer this question, and there were indeed some very definite answers.

What we're speaking of is named the specific dynamic action of foods. When you eat your protein, carbohydrate, and fat, each of them goes through a very different process of digestion, and before any of them are assimilated into your body to be used for growth or repair, or fuel, or to be stored as fat, your system must burn up a certain amount of energy (calories) to do the work of converting them into a more usable form. Just as you burn up a certain number of calories when you run for the bus, your body burns up a certain amount in making your food available to you. Scientists through experimentation discovered very early that protein burns up so much energy (as compared to carbohydrate and fat) in the process of digestion and assimilation that you get only a fraction of the protein calories that went into your mouth. The rest of the protein calories are used up in making it suitable for you to use. One of these researchers declared in 1969 that protein used up five times as many calories as did carbohydrate in providing its calories to the body, and seven times as much as fat. Here was a rationale for those diets that seemed to advocate virtually unlimited intake of meat.

The interesting thing about the specific dynamic action concept is that it died. Most theories become extinct when new concepts prove them wrong. We realize we've made errors in the past and once we investigate things with new and improved methods, we find that we've drawn the wrong conclusions. Not so in the case of the specific dynamic action of protein. As a concept, it simply died. Somewhere early in the last half of the twentieth century, scientists seem to have lost interest. They went off in other directions. I find this most interesting. Here we had a viable concept to explain a problem that had been needling us for years, and researchers just turned their backs on it in wholesale numbers. Today, you still see it referred to in the literature from time to time, but only by esoteric scientists studying other organisms. I rarely find even a mention of specific dynamic action when considering human nutrition.

In the early 1900s a Norwegian explorer by the name of Stefansson seemed to have become obsessed with convincing the world that the only diet for the human race was meat and fat. He had been shipwrecked and lived among Canadian Eskimos for one winter. He observed that they as well as he thrived on that kind of diet. When he got back to civilization he spent the better part of a year participating in a famous experiment where he and another man ate only meat and fat. The result certainly supported his position. He promoted his ideas in his many books, and in one, *The Fat of the Land,* the preface was authored by the most renowned cardiologist of our time, Dr. Paul Dudley White. Dr. White's name was a household word at that time. He was the doctor who tended to President Eisenhower when he had his heart attack.

My preference for high-protein diets for weight loss comes from my own experience. Over the years I have used a variety of diets on my patients. I've seen the results of each firsthand. I've learned a lot. It's the kind of learning that can't come from reading books or scientific papers. I've seen what doesn't work, what works a little, and what works very well. I, of course, go for the best result. The bottom line: *Consistently, my patients do better on high-protein diets.*

In Chapter 11 you will learn the details of the kind of diet I believe has the best chance of helping you lose your weight quickly, comfortably, and safely. I assume that you won't be surprised to learn that it is a high-protein diet.

For more on protein, see Appendix B.

Summing Up

• High-protein diets have been the standard for losing weight since the middle of the nineteenth century.
• The trend continued for at least 100 years.
• It was followed by a move toward much more carbohydrate, much less protein, and low fat, and during that period obesity has probably become more prevalent.
• The pendulum now seems to be swinging back to the high-protein type of diet for weight loss.
• The author has seen the high-protein approach as the most viable type of diet for controlling hunger and achieving the objective.

10

Cholesterol and Hypothyroidism

In the last chapter I explained my partiality to high-protein diets for my patients who are in the process of losing weight. We all equate protein with meat, and to many of us meat conjures up the evil specter of cholesterol and its partner in crime, saturated fat.

If you're fifty years old or younger, you probably can't remember a time when cholesterol wasn't a hot topic.

I probably took first notice of cholesterol in 1953, when a doctor by the name of Ancel Keys reported on the relationship between the level of cholesterol in the bloodstream and the incidence of coronary heart disease. I was still in medical school then, but when I first began my practice, I took up the banner like most practicing physicians and became an advocate of prudent eating. This meant that my patients had to cut way down on foods that contained saturated fats and cholesterol.

The information seemed to be clear enough. A busy doctor doesn't have time to research every new report. He must have some faith in what he is told. And, in this case, he was told plenty. It seems that the media has always had a love affair with the subject of cholesterol. Cholesterol isn't just the buzzword of recent decades; it's been a really hot topic since the fifties.

Like all practitioners, I read my share of papers in medical journals, but they were just a fragment of what was available to read. The popular press influences medical judgment perhaps as much as does the serious literature. When your doctor receives a daily barrage from the media of well-meaning advice on how to lower one's cholesterol, it has to influence what he tells his patients.

I tend to go overboard when I'm involved in a cause, and so I suspect that my efforts to convince my patients of the proper course of diet were probably more extreme than the average doctor's. I told them to cut down on animal fats, reduce dairy products drastically—in short, to be prudent. "The prudent diet" was around for years. I still hear references to it.

The cholesterol subject got a shot in the arm in the form of a nicely packaged set of materials, led by an impressive book labeled *Report of the Expert Panel on Detection, Evaluation, and Treatment of High Blood Cholesterol in Adults,* sent to me and to every other doctor in the country in 1988 by the National Heart, Lung, and Blood Institute, which was a division of the U.S. Department of Health and Human Services. You've got to show some respect for anything you receive adorned with such an impressive bunch of words, especially when it is put together so colorfully and professionally. Furthermore, it was full of names of every important medical school and hospital you could think of. This package wasn't the usual junk mail that doctors receive and which they promptly chuck into the wastebasket. This gift was from our government.

Here was an organized dissertation of the whole cholesterol story. It included a bit of history, instruction on how to evaluate your patients as to who in the population was at risk, a section on dietary treatment, and a segment on drug treatment of high cholesterol.

This was clearly a set of instructions designed for me to follow in my practice. The implication was unmistakable: Thou shalt do this. These were orders from above. It was my solemn duty as a physician to carry out this program.

With so much hype for the government's cause, it was about time for me to learn what this cholesterol business was all about. Of course I read the government materials, and they certainly made a good case for my pursuing their goals. Cholesterol did seem to be the killer and saturated fats its accomplice. Still, in the back of my brain was this disturbing feeling that there had been some alternative views of the whole thing. I couldn't even remember from what quarters these diverse thoughts came, but I decided to bone up on the subject. That was a few years back, but I've never lost interest in the project.

I have learned that the dissent over the importance of controlling one's cholesterol isn't trivial, even though it comes from a relatively small number of individuals and they don't seem to have the clout to get their message across.

Possibly, the first piece of dissent I ever read was a book by a Dr. Edward R. Pinckney, titled *Cholesterol Controversy,* written in 1973, fourteen years before the government really got that interested. He pointed out that the link between heart disease and cholesterol was simply not proved. He accused government agencies of having "allowed health associations and food industries to play havoc with the anxieties of millions and millions of people by permitting this unproved doctrine to be promoted."

A number of others have expressed similar doubts since that time, and a few books have been written on the subject. A 1989 article in the *Atlantic Monthly* titled "The Cholesterol Myth" fueled the controversy. The author, Thomas J. Moore, certainly suggested that a conspiracy involving the food industry, the drug industry, and government cooperation was out to deceive the public into believing stories about the villain cholesterol.

He was joined by others. A man by the name of Russell Smith did a tremendous amount of research in collecting everything known on the subject, came to the same conclusions, and presented his findings in a 1991 book. The controversy has since cooled somewhat, and even those who believe that the whole subject has been taken too seriously seem to be willing to play it safe by at least following dietary guidelines that purport to keep cholesterol under control.

Of course, we now know that there is "good" cholesterol and "bad" cholesterol and that we really don't mind when the former is elevated. In fact, a high level of good cholesterol, HDL, is said to be protective against cardiovascular disease. The scope of this book doesn't include an in-depth look at the whole cholesterol question. As a result, please assume that when I speak of high cholesterol, I'm referring to the alleged negative effects from elevated cholesterol that necessarily includes the bad part.

I have seen my share of high cholesterol readings. That isn't surprising when you consider that all of my patients come to me weighing more than they should. It is also expected that as the patient loses weight, the cholesterol will fall. The low-saturated-fat diet I prescribe for my patients is one factor promoting this. The weight loss itself contributes to lowering the cholesterol, as does the exercise prescription the patient is given.

Of my patients who are shown to be hypothyroid, cholesterol levels are higher than in those who don't have thyroid problems. That is one of the many indications that cause me to suspect hypothyroidism. Every new patient is required to have some routine laboratory testing, and cholesterol tests are included. I'm not sure if it is safe to say that every single "untreated" hypothyroid patient I have ever seen had an elevated cholesterol, but I really don't think I can remember an exception. When I see high cholesterol, I immediately think of hypothyroidism.

It is a rather general rule that as my patients lose weight, the cholesterol levels fall. This is even true of those whose cholesterol levels are normal at the onset. There is quite a range of what is considered normal cholesterol levels, so a drop doesn't take them out of the normal range.

In those patients I've diagnosed with hypothyroidism, the drop in cholesterol values once they've been placed on thyroid hormone treatment is more dramatic. The cholesterol lowering seems to take place in advance of what would have been attributed to weight loss. Many of these were previously aware of high cholesterol readings and have been admonished by their doctors to stop eating fat and to lose weight. Others have been put on cholesterol-lowering drugs, which did seem to have some beneficial effect. In spite of this, it is rare for me to see an obese patient who has achieved a normal cholesterol through the use of cholesterol-lowering medications. The cholesterol may have dropped, but it was still somewhat elevated.

On the other hand, treatment with thyroid hormone has resulted in many patients getting their cholesterol levels into the normal range, sometimes in conjunction with the other medications, but frequently without any other medication. It is commonplace for my hypothyroid patients to control their cholesterol readings totally through the use of thyroid hormone. They are always delighted when I take them off the cholesterol-lowering drugs. For one thing, these prescriptions are very expensive. These patients also know that there is some concern over liver damage from use of these drugs, and they welcome not having to have blood tests to monitor this possibility.

Unlike my disdain for thyroid testing of the blood, I have no cause to believe that cholesterol testing is inaccurate. Needless to say, I've done thousands of those tests also, and I'm quite satisfied that they are consistent and useful.

My purpose in including this chapter is to alert you to the possibility that if your cholesterol is found to be high, this could be useful information and it might very well point your doctor in the direction of suspecting hypothyroidism. Unfortunately, I believe that this particular finding is frequently overlooked. The drug companies have done a good job of convincing the practicing physician that they have the answer to the cholesterol problem and that writing the correct prescription for their products will do it.

If you choose to take the MFI test described in the next chapter and the result indicates that you could have a problem with hypothyroidism and you know your cholesterol is also elevated, it is time for action.

I believe you should diplomatically introduce the subject of your high cholesterol and its possible relationship to the thyroid when you visit your doctor. You could say, "Doctor, I read somewhere that high cholesterol is sometimes related to thyroid problems. Do you think that applies to me?" How is that for being subtle? You don't want to offend your doctor, but it's your body and your life. Act accordingly.

I believe that proper treatment of your low thyroid function can be a major step in lowering your cholesterol. Whether you're from the camp that accepts the current attitude toward cholesterol or are more attuned to those who question it, there is probably no harm in playing it safe. Proper treatment of your thyroid problem would be expected to lower your cholesterol levels, and your doctor will certainly be pleased with that result.

So far we've explored the thyroid and how its underactivity can affect your well-being. You've learned that the problem is often missed or ignored and why. We've delved into how hypothyroidism is treated. We have an inkling of the kind of diet that will reduce your weight, whether you have a thyroid problem or not. And you know there is a test you can give to yourself that could change your life. Now, let's get to it.

Summing Up

- The blood cholesterol level is usually elevated in those with hypothyroidism.
- The role of elevated blood cholesterol as a cause of heart disease is questioned by some authorities.
- Thyroid-related elevated cholesterol often responds to treatment with thyroid hormone without resorting to other cholesterol-lowering drugs.

11
The Metabolic Function Index Test

It's time to get down to business.

You're about to test your metabolism. That's essentially another way of saying that you will be testing your thyroid. But that may not be exactly correct either. What we're really testing is whether your body is supplying itself with enough thyroid hormone. From a practical standpoint, it is all the same thing. The nuances of how we play with the words have little to do with the actual goal of this exercise. We're about to find out whether you burn up enough calories, and if you don't, you will find out what you can do about it.

You indeed may be someone who is already taking a prescription for thyroid hormone. If that is the case, it will probably be for levothyroxine, T4, but there is always the possibility that your doctor, like me, prefers to prescribe natural thyroid. The test you will perform has value whether you are known to have hypothyroidism or you have undiscovered hypothyroidism. It is even valuable if you don't have hypothyroidism. In that event, it will tell you that you don't need hormone replacement therapy and that a reduced-calorie diet will have you losing weight like all those "normal" people do.

If you're currently taking some form of thyroid, natural or synthetic, the test will serve as a check on whether you're receiving the right amount. It will inform you whether the amount of thyroid hormone you're taking is sufficient to cause you to burn calories at a normal rate. Remember, I've indicated that the most revealing sign of hypothyroidism is the inadequate burning of calories. This test will reveal whether the added thyroid you're taking brings your metabolism into the normal range. It may serve to inform you that you need more thyroid hormone.

The theory behind the test you will be performing on yourself is based upon how you handle food energy in comparison to a theoretically normal person with your same characteristics. When it is completed you will know how you stack up against that "normal" individual.

The normalcy we're investigating is limited to how you process energy. You will recall that we use the word *energy* rather loosely in this book as synonymous with *calories* or perhaps even *food*. That's where we get our energy, from food. This is the scientists' use of the word *energy*. It isn't the popular usage, where energy may mean pep or enthusiasm or stamina. The word *calorie* is actually a unit of energy, just as the pound is a unit of weight or the inch is a unit of length.

Picture an imaginary person whom we shall call our *model*. Of course, if you're to compare yourself to some normal model, we must know something about that model. We want the model to have your physical characteristics. A major part of the calculation you will make later on is aimed at defining this model or normal person.

Here, briefly, is what the task entails: We will be looking at someone with your same height, weight, age, and activity level, and we're going to determine how many calories that model requires each day to maintain his or her weight. Suppose with our calculations we were to come up with 2,150 calories. That would mean that a "normal" model individual with your same characteristics would neither lose weight nor gain weight on a diet of 2,150 calories per day. We shall call this our standard caloric maintenance level and for convenience will abbreviate it as the SCML.

The test takes twenty-eight days to complete, but your task during those twenty-eight days is little more than to follow a particular diet for that period of time. The diet is a 1,000-calorie diet that will certainly result in weight loss even in the reader with the most severe hypothyroidism. The tables you will consult and the few calculations you will make at the conclusion of the diet period are based on staying on the diet for twenty-eight days. They will have no validity if you stop the diet earlier. Let's approach this test seriously, with all the fervor of a mad scientist. The information you will gain will be very valuable to you. You will discover how your metabolism compares with the norm. You will know what it takes for you to lose weight. You may answer the perplexing question of why it has been difficult for you to lose weight or maintain weight. Don't treat this casually. You have a task ahead of you. Not a difficult one, but a serious one.

The 1,000-calorie diet may not be that different from other low-calorie diets you've tried in the past. It isn't particularly difficult to follow. It is designed for convenience. After all these years of treating overweight patients, I'm well aware of the time constraints that plague many of my patients. It offers the convenience of prepared packaged meals from the supermarket as an alternative to cooking up a storm.

Will the test cut into your busy schedule? Absolutely not. Aside from the requirement to eat according to the instructions, your other tasks should take less than three minutes a day. You need only to record your weight on the first day and then again on the twenty-ninth day. There is a two-minute task you will perform before your day actually begins, indeed, before you even get out of bed. The largest task will be to use the tables and to make the necessary calculations. That all happens at the end of the twenty-eight-day diet.

As valuable as my MFI test should be to my patients, there are always a few who simply will not comply sufficiently for four straight weeks so that I can get a valid reading of their metabolism. Immediately, Lucy comes to mind.

Lucy was five feet four inches tall and weighed 263 pounds. Those figures spell danger. Everyone who laid eyes on her had to be aware that she was in big trouble. Lucy told me right from the first that she had a thyroid problem. She had been tested several times, but had rejected what the doctors told her. She knew she had a thyroid problem and she wasn't ashamed to tell me about it. She wasn't angry with her former doctors. She wasn't the type to be angry with anyone.

"I don't eat that much, but I do have a yen for candy. I play cards with my friends three times a week and there is always candy. I just can't resist." In spite of this, Lucy was adamant that her diet didn't account for her bulk.

She had various other symptoms that tended to confirm her own diagnosis. If I had been forced to make a yes or no guess at that moment, it would have been an emphatic yes. I told her that I felt she was probably hypothyroid and would most likely benefit from taking thyroid hormone, but first we needed to confirm it. I told her about the MFI test. Her attitude: "Let's go."

Four weeks later, I learned that the test was marred by several social events that occurred during the month. She had tried, but she had lost nothing. Absolutely nothing. That told me a lot. Hypothyroidism or not, "nothing" isn't an option. She apologized and said that next month she would adhere and I would get the information I needed.

I recall that the next month wasn't much better; Lucy lost only a pound or two. In an extreme case that could have been valid, but she freely admitted her indiscretions. She asked me to prescribe thyroid hormone anyway, appealing to my sympathy. She said she could hardly make it through her day and she needed that act of mercy. She knew all about thyroid treatment, and my usual lecture wasn't needed. I did lecture her on the necessity of giving me one good month so that I could confirm her problem. Lucy promised she'd try again.

She broke her promise. The months that followed were each like an instant replay. I would emphasize the necessity for one good month of 800 calories a day, she would entreat me to give her the thyroid, I would refuse, and she would promise again. Would you believe that this went on for over a year? She lost only thirteen pounds for the whole year, not enough to matter at all.

Finally, I got tough. I told her that this game we were playing was ridiculous. I suggested that there was no point in her going on. This was nothing new to me. I've had to do that with patients many times. I was being honest, but at the same time I knew she would end up going to another doctor or "clinic" and wouldn't do any better. I wanted her to stay with me, but I also wanted results. The only way to really help Lucy was to force her into action. My veiled threat of giving up on her worked. The next month, I got what I wanted. She had lost five pounds and I felt certain she was being honest.

You, like Lucy, must be honest, but with yourself. If you momentarily stray from the diet, you won't have to worry about my reprimanding you. If you stray, you must honestly record your indiscretions on the Excess Calorie Sheet.

When the four weeks are over, the final task shouldn't take more than fifteen minutes. A pocket calculator could help if you don't feel like multiplying.

Let's begin.

On page 161 you will find the MFI Calculation Form. On the morning you're to start your diet, you must weigh yourself. This should be done before eating or drinking anything and after you've completed your morning bathroom functions. You will be weighing yourself again at the end of the twenty-eight days. What is important is that both weighings be done under identical conditions. You may want to use your own bathroom scale if you know that it is reasonably accurate. Otherwise, look for a good scale. Perhaps a friend has a doctor's scale, one of those where you slide the weights around. I've seen high-quality scales in supermarkets. Ideally you would want your nude weight both at the beginning and at the end. This can be accomplished even if you use the scale in your supermarket. Bear with me. It can be done. I promise you will not be arrested in the act.

Your Nude Weight

The easiest way to do this is to get on the scale while you're naked as a jaybird. That could prove inconvenient if you're weighing yourself in a public place. But there is a way. You must know the weight of the clothing you're wearing and then subtract it from what you weigh clothed. I'm speaking of the weight of all of the clothing, every last item. Even if your home scale isn't accurate enough to weigh you, it should be good enough to weigh your clothing. Don't weigh your clothes by placing them on the scale. That won't work. Here is how you do it.

At home, weigh yourself while wearing specific clothes. Mark down the weight. Now remove all the clothes, step on the scale, and weigh yourself nude. Mark down your nude weight. Subtract the second weight from the first. The difference is the weight of your clothes. Armed with that information, you may now go to some accurate scale and weigh yourself while wearing those exact same clothes. Subtract the weight of your clothes. That is your nude weight. Now wasn't that easy?

If it isn't possible to obtain your nude weight, you will have to estimate the weight of your clothes and subtract it from your dressed weight. If you choose to do this, take the time to indicate exactly what you were wearing at the time of the weighing. Note everything: outer clothes, underwear, the particular pair of shoes, etc. You will want to wear the exact same outfit when you do your final weighing. The more precise you are, the more reliable the result.

There is another little task you must do before you begin the test. I want you to take your temperature. This should be the first thing you do on the day you start the diet, in fact it should be done while you're still in bed, before you've walked around, before you've brushed your teeth, before you've had your coffee. You must therefore prepare for it the night before. There should be a thermometer on the night table next to your bed, already shaken down and ready for use. Pop it into your mouth, under your tongue, as soon as you awaken. Leave it in for about two minutes. Write down the result next to the first date on the Daily Temperature Chart on page 174.

Please buy yourself a glass thermometer for a couple of bucks if you don't already have one. These are the ones with the thin shiny column of mercury inside. Don't worry. The mercury won't harm you as long as it remains on the inside. Some of the results from the newer gadgets are questionable. I believe that your temperature is best taken in your mouth and not in your ear. So take your temperature, write it down, shake down the thermometer, and get it ready for the next day. You will need to take your temperature most mornings for those twenty-eight days and record these readings on the chart. Don't forget to do it before you get out of bed. If you forget and remember later, don't take your temperature that day. Leave that day blank on the Daily Temperature Chart. Try not to miss too many days. I would like to see at least fifteen readings for the twenty-eight days. For females, don't record temperatures on the days during menstruation. In fact, to play it safe, exclude the day before and the day after also.

Of course, such daily temperature readings won't be valid if you're ill during the test. If you have a cold or other infection, there is no point in recording those temperature readings on the chart. Then again, if you're really sick, you will probably not be performing the test during that time. So pick a time when you're healthy, and start again.

Your intention is (I hope) to follow the 1,000-calorie diet to the letter, but it is possible that you may slip up a bit. I hope these distractions will be infrequent. Nonetheless, we don't want the whole test to be abandoned just because you weakened on a few occasions. You will still have a valid test if you have prepared for that possibility in advance. Put aside a sheet of paper that you've labeled "Excess Calories for the 28 Days." Make two columns, one for the date, and one for the excess calories for that particular date. As the test proceeds, write in the dates when you exceeded the 1,000-calorie allowance, and next to each jot down your estimate of how many extra calories (above 1,000) you ate that day. To repeat, don't count all the calories that day, only the amount over 1,000. At the end of the twenty-eight days, add up all the excess calories. You will need this number when it comes to calculating your MFI.

A variation on this test is described in Appendix C. It explains how to adjust the 1,000 calories per day to a higher amount and still have a valid test.

Of course, in order to do this, you must have a means of estimating how many calories were in that hamburger you just had. This can be hard to do, or not so hard, depending on how prepared you are. If it happens in one of the fast-food franchises, you can often get the information right there. They may have posted their nutritional information or the clerk may be able to help you. If the excess occurs as the result of eating some packaged food, the answer will probably be on the nutritional chart on the package. If it occurs at home or at a friend's house or at a street-vendor's hot dog cart, you will need to consult one of the excellent "calorie books" that are around. See Appendix G.

If you never deviate (an inspiring thought), you don't have to buy one of those books, but it is always wise to be prepared for the unexpected.

Here is what your Excess Calorie List might look like:

Excess Calories for the 28 Days

June	23	240
	28	220
July	4	750
	9	125
	10	340
	11	50
	16	210
		1,935

Now it's time to begin the diet. Go to Chapter 12 for the details.

Summing Up

- The Metabolic Function Index test provides the convenient and accurate means for assessing the adequacy of the rate at which the individual burns calories.
- The twenty-eight-day test can be performed on oneself at home.
- The accuracy of the test depends upon the care that is exerted in following the instructions.
- Two other corroborating tests will also be furnished.
- A high-protein diet is encouraged as a means of controlling hunger during the test.

12
How to Test Yourself

This diet is the test diet that you will follow for the twenty-eight days of the test. If it then seems advisable (to be discussed later), you will continue with the very same diet as your weight-loss diet. This is the diet to follow until you've achieved your proper weight.

There has been a lot of controversy over the years around how to determine what an ideal weight should be. Various authorities will give more or less importance to such factors as height, age, and bone structure. Information derived from publications of the Metropolitan Life Insurance Company has been among the most accepted during this century, though even these sources weren't free of criticism. The BBW (baseline body weight) table on page 166 should serve as a guide, although it was intended as a baseline for the later calculation of your Metabolic Function Index. You may use it as a general guide of what you should weigh, but realize that there is no such thing as an exact proper weight. This particular table doesn't take into consideration such things as frame size and age, but those will be factored into our calculations later. You may consider 5 percent above or below the given weight acceptable.

The essential requirements of any diet that is to be followed

over a period of time are threefold: effectiveness, safety, and convenience. We might focus on safety as the most important of
these, but in a sense they share rather equal importance since each
is essential if the program is to be a success. I've endeavored, here
and in my practice, to present a set of instructions that embraces
those three elements.

Effectiveness

The statement that follows may seem a bit smug. *You will lose
weight on this diet.* How can I be so sure of myself? It's simple:
Everyone loses weight on a 1,000-calorie diet. That's even more smug,
but I have equal confidence in that one. In some cases the loss
might seem to be painfully slow and meager. If that is the case,
the explanation for this will seem clearer when you examine the
results of the MFI test. If you have any degree of hypothyroidism,
the weight loss will be less than expected. Indeed, that is why you
will suspect hypothyroidism; it is because the weight loss is inadequate. No matter how meager, you will lose something on a
diet of 1,000 calories per day. No one has a metabolism that low.

Safety

I'm often asked whether the weight-loss diet I prescribe for my
patients is a proper diet. The answer is always no. This answer
usually results in eyebrows being raised, and they don't really
come down again until I have completed my explanation: "No, it
isn't proper. A proper diet doesn't result in weight loss, nor does
it result in weight gain. By its very definition, a proper diet results in what will maintain you at a proper weight and in good
health, and permanently to boot. If you are to lose weight, the
diet must necessarily be improper."

If I still have the patient's attention, I go on. "To lose weight
you must eat fewer calories than your body burns. For the most
part, the greater the deficiency you create, the faster the weight

loss. Once you've achieved your normal weight, we can then shift our attention to a proper diet."

Of course this is just a bit of verbal gymnastics, but it does help to get my point across. If we want to elaborate on the use of the word *proper,* I may then add that the diet they've been given is indeed a *proper* diet for losing weight.

The diet that is specified in these pages isn't the exact diet I use with my patients. The difference is in the number of calories per day. The diet you will be following for the MFI test supplies 1,000 calories per day. Later, with the help of your doctor, you may be placed on a few more calories per day, although in some instances, perhaps it will be a few less. By contrast, in my own practice I use an 800-calorie diet and I'm quite comfortable in doing so. I have a wealth of information that shows me that patients do quite well on that number of calories and that surprisingly few problems arise. Of course, my patients are seen very frequently and are monitored very closely. Since you aren't my patient and I will not be personally checking you, I'm more comfortable with your getting a few more calories per day, if your doctor approves, and I do feel strongly that you should make a few visits to your doctor during those four weeks just to be sure everything is going well. My own patients are seen weekly during that period. The MFI test you will be taking is based upon your following a 1,000-calorie diet for four weeks, and all the calculations are based upon those numbers.

A variation of this test is described in Appendix C. It explains how to adjust the 1,000 calories per day to a higher amount and still have a valid test.

Convenience

Let's face it, if a diet you are given puts too much of a burden on you, if it is too much in conflict with your lifestyle, you will probably abandon it. In fact, you may already have done just that enough times in the past. Remember, virtually any diet that comes from a magazine or from a book will result in weight loss if—here is where the big IF comes in—*if you follow the diet.* Have you ever declared, "I wasn't able to follow that diet"?

The likelihood of remaining on a diet decreases as the time spent on it increases. In my own experience, those who successfully achieve their weight goal do it quickly. Those who frequently falter along the way and thus prolong the time required are more apt to abandon the effort. This also seems to apply to "maintenance diets." How many people gain back the weight in spite of the seemingly proper maintenance diet advocated by one of these diet clinics or organizations! Was it because the long-term diet they had been given was improper? No, I don't think so. The diet would have worked to maintain weight if the dieters had followed it. There's the rub! They didn't follow it.

This also seems to be the rule in my medical practice. If I give a patient a lifetime diet (which I have in the past), I know it will be followed for a while—a week, a month, or even a year. But eventually the patient will get away from it, particularly if the office visits have come to a halt, and I will generally see that person again when the decision to lose weight kicks in once more. That is why I've developed a rather unconventional approach to weight maintenance.

Convenience in a diet necessarily means that the diet is practical; it is one that can be followed in the course of the usual day's activities. I tend to personalize such things and present a diet in terms of what would suit my own needs. I'm a busy guy, much like most of my patients. I suspect that with the help of a few professional chefs I could write a cookbook that would meet the specifications of the type of diet I would really prefer for my readers. They could then spend the day acquiring a whole host of ingredients, dumping them in the kitchen, and then putting in their time at the stove cooking up a storm. If the quantities served fell within the guidelines, they could even lose weight while dining on succulent meals. But is that a practical option for the majority of people? Have I not heard of a celebrity who acquired a personal chef to ensure that her weight-losing experience wasn't too painful?

With a rare exception, my patients must seek more practical means.

Practicality means convenience, and the diet that follows is geared to convenience. I've minimized the time spent in the kitchen. Anything that speeds up the process of providing the food is considered a plus. A microwave could help immensely. At least during the twenty-eight-day period of the test, I think you might also want to dispense with the trappings that make dining such a pleasure. The fine china, the lace tablecloth, the dimmed lights, the candelabra, and the dinner music all seem to favor an eating orgy rather than a weight-loss meal. In short, eat what you're supposed to and get it over with. Let's save the fine dining for some future time.

Your goal will be to eat 1,000 calories a day of a diet very high in protein, with a moderate amount of carbohydrate, and a relatively small amount of fat. A common dietary recommendation is that 30 percent of our calories come from fat and 55 to 60 percent from carbohydrates. That leaves but 10 to 15 percent from protein. As you've read here, I can't go along with that distribution for a weight-loss diet. I like protein for weight loss. We're going to reduce your fat intake to no more than 25 percent and increase the protein all the way up to at least 28 percent. That will leave the carbohydrates supplying about 47 percent of your calories. Remember, these values are for the percentage of calories that come from each of the three groups. This doesn't translate directly into the weight of food in each group. That last statement may sound confusing, but you don't have to dwell on it. Remember not to use those figures in searching for food. I will give you very good guidelines for that task. The diet itself will specify quantities of foods that will result in the above distribution so that you will not have to worry about what percentage of this or that is in what you're eating.

Could you eat more protein and less of the other two? Yes. I would even prefer it. The problem with that is practicality. I have already spoken of convenience. The availability of a higher-protein diet than I've settled for could be the stumbling block.

Were I to insist upon higher protein and less fat and carbohydrate, virtually no frozen dinners would be acceptable.

The closer you come to supplying the 1,000 calories a day, the more accurate will be the result you obtain in calculating your MFI. In spite of this, I don't consider exact adherence to the specified foods and quantities a cast-in-stone requirement. That may seem inconsistent, but I'll explain why it isn't. What really counts is that you eat 1,000 calories per day. How you get to that number is somewhat less important. The main reason for following my instructions exactly is that the job will be easier. Specifically, you will be less hungry than if the distribution of nutrients is altered. If you're a total maverick and choose your own 1,000-calorie mix, as long as you're accurate, I expect the bottom line to be acceptable. You can do it your way, but I'll bet you will be less hungry and more comfortable if you do it my way.

Emphasis on Protein

This is a high-protein diet, perhaps not as high in protein as some of the bizarre diets currently circulating, but high enough to accomplish its purpose. If we ignore the specific dynamic action of protein that I spoke of in an earlier chapter, we can get down to this subject of eating protein for hunger control. After years of addressing my patients' struggles with hunger, I'm convinced that an abundance of protein keeps hunger manageable, but a little carbohydrate—surprisingly little—can make you ravenous. Like other advice in this book, this observation is based upon experience. The counterpart of this canon is that when patients confess to deviating from my recommendations, when they overdo carbohydrates at the expense of protein, they report an uncomfortable degree of hunger that causes them to eat more calories than are allowed. When patients really complain that the diet doesn't satisfy hunger, it is often difficult for me to pry out of them honest information about what they've been eating. I must often probe relentlessly until I secure the admission that this person complaining of hunger has been eating bread or drinking orange juice or using enough breath mints to deodorize a regiment.

What I've reported aren't theoretical concepts that come from an institutionally sponsored study or from work on laboratory animals. This information is admittedly "anecdotal." But it does come from real people, thousands of them, earnestly seeking the help of their doctor.

Breakfast

One of the more common problems with low-calorie diets is constipation. Without getting into the semantics involved, the complaint that I hear so often may not be constipation at all, but rather infrequent bowel movements. Let's get right to the issue. You will not have the same bowel movements when you're eating 1,000 calories a day as when you were eating 3,000 calories a day. There is simply not enough bulk and generally much less fiber for that to happen. The fact that your bowel movements often skip a day or two may not literally be constipation, but whatever name it is called, it is distressing to most dieters. I generally draw the line at what makes my patient physically uncomfortable. If this infrequency causes real physical discomfort, it is time for action. Of course, the best course of action is prevention.

What does breakfast have to do with it? For the most part, we're going to solve this troublesome problem at breakfast. Breakfast is going to be a cereal, and preferably one with a good amount of dietary fiber. That should essentially solve the problem of constipation. Choose the ½ cup (1 oz.) serving size of the one below or experiment with others. There is a simple way to boost the fiber content of any cereal and nullify the constipating effect of low-calorie eating: Add bran. A good choice comes in a jar. Add a heaping tablespoonful of Kretschmer Toasted Wheat Germ to your cereal. It will boost the calories by only about 15, but will add 3 grams of fiber.

If you choose cereals other than the one below, look for those that have 180 calories or less (without the milk) per 2-ounce serving. Use milk with it (2 percent fat is desirable), but there is no point in using more than you need, since it does have about 16 calories per ounce. Use just enough milk to wet the cereal. There is no need to slosh it on. Be aware of how many ounces of milk you have used. As a breakfast beverage, you may have a cup of coffee or tea, or if you're one of those addicts, a diet soda is acceptable. If you must lighten your coffee, use milk with 2 percent fat. Don't forget to count its calories into your day's total. I like the following best because of the low calories:

Calories per Ounce

Kellogg's All-Bran with Extra Fiber	54

Lunch

The extent to which your lunch contributes to the day's 1,000 calories is a matter of personal preference. You will have a lot of leeway. It doesn't matter particularly whether lunch or dinner is the "main" meal. I even see a fair amount of patients who insist that they never have lunch. If you're comfortable with that, it's okay. It will necessarily allow you to have a bigger dinner, a requirement that should not be too distressing to you. My medical practice is now principally in South Florida, where there is a predominantly Latin influence. In most of the Latin countries, the midday meal is the main meal, and this diet could easily be varied to accommodate that as well as other cultural preferences. Again, the bottom line is 1,000 calories; when you eat them is less important.

Dinner

The majority of readers will probably choose to have their main meal in the evening. As you would expect, the food choices that follow are designed to slant the diet in the direction of protein. Carbohydrates will generally be from those that are the more complex, and fat will be minimal. A little arithmetic will be required to add up the day's calories. You must come as close to 1,000 as possible. You could probably do quite well simply by using the calorie values specified in this chapter, but if you want to expand into foods that I haven't included, you will need the help of one of the better "calorie books." I have recommended some of these in Appendix G.

Frozen dinners are particularly convenient, and you may want to use them frequently. They may be eaten for lunch as well. Just keep track of the calories. The frozen dinners I've selected and which are listed later in this chapter are particularly desirable because of their distribution of nutrients. You may use others that aren't on the list, but try not to deviate too often. As a bonus for following my recommendations and availing yourself of the listed foods, I believe you will have the least problem with hunger.

Snacks

I'm certainly not encouraging you to have snacks during the test. The typical snack that comes in those gloriously colorful bags is certainly not advised. Yet one positive purpose for a snack is to make up for not eating enough calories that day. If by evening your total for the day is 900 calories, you should supplement that day's intake with 100 calories of something. I'm not suggesting that you order a pizza. Choose something from the lists provided.

Packaged Foods and Frozen Foods

I like frozen foods because they work for my patients. Busy people particularly like the convenience of the whole meal in a box. Once they understand what is available and which of them suits their tastes, they do well with these single meals in a box. They share the advantages of other packaged products in that you know exactly what you're getting in terms of calories. You don't need a calorie book. It's all there on the nutritional panel. I have listed some of the frozen foods I've evaluated. I didn't choose them from those mouthwatering pictures on the box or even from the taste; I haven't tasted many of them. The selection process had only to do with the nutritional information supplied to me by the manufacturer or that I copied directly from the nutritional panel on the package. Like my other food choices, you will note that the products listed have more protein and less fat for the amount of calories they supply than many other products that didn't make it onto my lists. Remember that all calorie counts in my frozen-meal lists are for one serving, an amount that is specified on the package. With most of these frozen dinners, a whole package constitutes a single serving.

There is considerable variation in the number of calories of the various frozen dinners I've chosen, but none is above 400 calories. You must take into account how each will fit in with your 1,000-calorie day. If you haven't had many calories by dinnertime, you should probably choose one that has a larger number of calories. You may even have to supplement your evening meal with something additional to reach the 1,000-calorie mark. This all takes planning, but it is worth the effort. You will acquire valuable information about yourself.

The Food Tables and Recommendations

The information I'm providing for you comes from the best sources available. With packaged foods, I've contacted the manufacturers, and if they were cooperative, I've used their information. Some of the data comes directly from the actual packages on supermarket shelves in various parts of the country. Some has been provided by restaurant chains. Much of it comes from the government. The United States Department of Agriculture maintains an enormous database of the nutritional makeup of foods in this country. I've used the latest version of this database to make my calculations.

With fresh food, things like fruits, vegetables, meats, and poultry, items that are loose or packaged by the supermarket and which don't have nutritional information, I've provided the calories per ounce, ignoring what is a normal serving. You will decide on the serving size and therefore how many calories that number of ounces contains. With that information, you can be very precise in supplying as many calories as you need to contribute to the 1,000 for the day. You will need a food scale for the test, but you can dispense with it for your remaining time on the diet.

Remember that my recommendations are based upon my experience, particularly as it relates to hunger, but don't consider them that rigid. Rather than abandon the diet and the test, you could go outside my recommendations. In the end the test will still be valid if you've kept track of the calories. As an example, were you to use the higher-calorie non-dairy creamers in your coffee, keep track of the calories and you will still be okay. But remember, if you squander your calories on such things, you will have less to allocate to "real" food.

In keeping with my preferences, I've only included information on those foods I recommend. If you go outside my choices, and you may, you will have to obtain the information from the food package.

With packaged foods, you will find that I've included only the more recognizable brand names, those that are generally available throughout the country. There are many lesser-known brands, regional brands, and house brands of supermarkets that are just as good. If the nutritional panel on the package becomes a habit, you won't go wrong.

I have listed my choices by rather loosely chosen alphabetized categories.

Sample Daily Menus

See Appendix I (pages 260–64).

Beef

Your selection of beef is limited, but you may indeed have beef. Choose cuts that have 5 percent or less of fat. The government grades beef by the amount of fat it contains. Whether you agree or not, the fattest is considered the best; the highest grade is U.S. Prime. For that reason, Prime isn't advisable for this diet. The next two lesser grades are Choice and Select, which have respectively less fat. There are grades below Select with even less fat, but they are quite tough unless cooked to death. Remember that the calories per ounce given below are for raw beef and you should make your calculations from that value. After cooking you will have fewer ounces, mainly because of water loss, but the calories will be changed very little.

Beef cut	Grade
Beef, round, full cut	Choice
Beef, round, eye round	Choice
Beef, round, tip round	Choice
Beef, round, top round	Choice
Beef, shank, cross-cuts	Choice
Beef, chuck, arm pot roast	Select
Beef, round, full cut	Select
Beef, round, bottom round	Select
Beef, round, eye of round	Select
Beef, round, top round	Select
Beef, short loin, top loin	Select
Beef, top sirloin	Select
Beef, short loin, T-bone steak	Select

What is supplied here is the latest information from our government. The names of the cuts are taken from the government's database. The calories are counted with beef trimmed to ¼ inch fat. You should eat the "separable lean only" part of the meat. The calories per ounce for each of the cuts above varies from 34 to 39, so you may make your calculations based upon a middle number of 37.

Ground beef deserves special mention. All of the prepackaged ground beef I've found in supermarkets contains too much fat. The lowest was marked extra-lean, but it still had 10 percent fat. If you must have ground beef, choose one of the acceptable cuts above and have the meat department grind it for you. That way it will satisfy the requirement.

Example: If you need a 225-calorie meat portion for dinner, use 6 ounces. Six times 37 is 222. That's close enough.

Beverages

I would like you to drink plenty of fluid, which really means water. Yet, in the end, whatever you drink is basically flavored water. Sometimes the "water" is combined with sugar and results in a lot of calories (juices, for example). For this test, let's forgo fruit juices and juice drinks even though they may be loaded with vitamins. Bubbly water such as seltzer and club soda are fine, but make sure the "seltzer" has no calories. I've seen flavored seltzers on the shelves that were high in calories. They were nothing more than the usual soda pop without the coloring agent. Bottled or canned soda pop should always be of the "diet" variety, and unless you have more than three a day, you don't need to count the calories.

There are some non-carbonated beverages you may wish to use. Crystal Light and sugar-free Kool-Aid each have 5 calories per 8-ounce glass.

Coffee and tea are also allowed. I've never observed caffeine to be a factor as far as weight loss is concerned. The problem arises with what you add to coffee or tea. Sugar should be out. Artificial sweeteners are allowed; they have virtually no calories. You should discipline yourself to add only low-fat milk with 2 percent fat to lighten coffee. Figure 15 calories per ounce, which is 2 tablespoonfuls. As to other "lighteners," they simply have too many calories, which you get at the expense of other good solid food. Given that you will have only 1,000 calories, you don't want to squander them. If you must, there are some fat-free non-dairy creamers with about 7 calories per ounce (2 tablespoonfuls). Their availability varies and is often regional. Check your supermarket, read the labels, and count the calories.

Regular unsweetened tea is fine, cold or hot, as are a number of "diet" teas. Lipton, for example, has several of them with 5 calories per 8-ounce glass. Don't forget to count those calories if you have three glasses or more per day.

Bread

Save it till you're thin. It's all carbohydrate. Have faith—you will be able to eat bread again.

Butter and Margarine

Of course not. All fat and way too many calories to waste. There are some pretty fair attempts at least to reproduce the flavor. I actually think the sprays are useful. Don't overdo them and you won't have to count their calories. Try these:

I Can't Believe It's Not Butter! Spray
Parkay Buttery Spray

There is also a spread, Fleischmann's fat-free 5-calorie spread, with that amount per tablespoonful.

Candies

I really can't find any I could recommend. Watch out for the so-called sugar-free variety. They are free of sugar only through a technicality. They may be sweetened with concentrated fruit juice, which is really just another name for sugar. (Baked goods also.) The calories on the label tell the story. The candies with sorbitol could keep you closer to the bathroom than you care to be.

Cheese

Most cheese is just too high in fat and therefore in calories for you even to consider it. There are some attempts to imitate the flavor of real cheeses, and you may experiment with them if you must. The label names can be very confusing, particularly because of the variety. Try to look for the names I've spelled out here and pay close attention to the nutritional panel on the package.

	Calories per Ounce
Kraft Free Singles American, Swiss, or Sharp Cheddar (1 slice)	30
Polly-O Free Natural Non-Fat Ricotta (⅛ cup)	25
Kraft Philadelphia Free Fat-Free Cream Cheese (several varieties)	30
Breakstone's Free Fat-Free Cottage Cheese	20
Light n' Lively Fat-Free Cottage Cheese	20

Chicken, Canned

There are a number of satisfactory varieties of lesser-known brands. On the label, the chicken should be listed at 60 calories per 2-ounce serving. Some have a few more calories than 30 per ounce. Try to stick to those with 30 per ounce. Here are some name brands:

	Calories per Ounce
Hormel Premium Chunk Breast of Chicken in Water	30
Swanson Premium Chunk White Chicken in Water	30

Crabmeat, Imitation

This is also called surimi. It is fish made to resemble crabmeat and flavored to simulate it. There are other varieties that imitate lobster. There are a number of brands, and they all seem to have between 26 and 30 calories per ounce. Surimi has more carbohydrate than I like, but you might want to give it a try.

Deli Meats

I recommend these because they are easy to come by and high in protein, just the thing for someone who is always on the run. I've eaten my share of them. In this instance, since the products are sliced, I specify the calories per slice as well as the calories per ounce. These types of products come in a variety of presentations and different-sized slices. Many more are acceptable than I've listed here. The following should give you a variety of choices.

Fat-Free Cold Cuts	Calories per Slice	Calories per Ounce
Louis Rich		
Turkey Breast, Oven Roasted	25	25
Turkey Breast, Hickory Smoked	25	25
Oven Roasted Breast of Turkey	25	25
Rotisserie Flavor Breast of Turkey	25	25
Chicken Breast, Oven Roasted Deluxe	30	30
Turkey Ham	30	30
Turkey Pastrami	30	30

Oscar Meyer

Ham, Baked Cooked	23	31
Ham, Boiled	20	27
Turkey, White, Oven Roasted	30	30
Canadian-Style Bacon	25	30

Hillshire Farm

Pastrami	10	30
Honey Ham	10	30

Hormel

Light & Lean 97 Sliced Ham	25	25
Sliced Mesquite Smoked Turkey		
Breast	30	30

Dressings

Be careful here. The fine reputation that salads enjoy as diet food is unwarranted when the dressing has a zillion calories. Look for 30 calories or less per ounce, which is usually specified as 2 tablespoonfuls. Be careful. The calories can mount up with these. Here are a few salad dressings:

	Calories per Ounce
Weight Watchers	
Creamy Italian	30
Caesar	10
Italian	10
Pritikin	
Dijon Balsamic Vinaigrette	30

Mayonnaise

The real stuff is out, but there are some pretty fair imitations. Remember that an ounce is about 2 tablespoonfuls. Try these:

	Calories per Ounce
Kraft Mayo Fat-Free	
Mayonnaise Dressing	10
Weight Watchers Whipped Dressing	15
Kraft Miracle Whip Free Dressing	15

Eggs

Unfortunately, whole eggs aren't acceptable because of the fat content of the yolk. By contrast, the white of the egg is about the highest-quality protein you can obtain, and it is virtually pure protein. A single egg white (from a large egg) adds about 18 calories. The difference in the calories in the egg white alone of eggs of different sizes is so minimal that you may ignore it and count 18 calories for any egg. You can do some creative things with egg white; you can blend it into a number of foods, such as vegetables, and it enhances them, particularly if you use some spices.

The "imitation" egg products are also quite good. They are essentially egg whites flavored to simulate whole eggs, and they have no fat and very little carbohydrate. I've listed some of the more popular brands. Don't forget to pay attention to the calories and include them in your daily total. Usually 2 ounces approximates one large egg.

	Calories per Ounce
Second Nature Fat-Free	13
Table Ready Real Egg	15
All Whites	13
Better 'n Eggs	14
Egg Beaters	15

Fish and Seafood

This category is perhaps the best "diet" food. It is high in protein and generally very low in carbohydrate. However, some varieties of fish (though not shellfish) are quite high in fat. Salmon is an example of an unacceptable fish for our purposes.

There are many choices of fish, and their availability may depend upon where you live. I've never even heard of some of the fish in the acceptable list I've compiled, but I've done my homework and I've given you the data. There may be some confusion inherent in the names of various fish. Striped bass is acceptable, but freshwater bass is not. Bluefin tuna has too much fat, but all the other varieties of tuna are just fine, including the canned variety (packed in water).

Virtually all shellfish may be eaten: crab, lobster, shrimp, clams, mussels, conch, etc. The trick is to know what quantity you will be eating. If you buy raw oysters or clams in the shell, you will need to weigh the edible portion while it is raw. This task could be more than you bargained for. Since there are so many other fish and seafood choices, you may choose to postpone the pleasure of eating some of these until after the test diet.

The list of fish I've provided is quite long. There are simply so many choices when it comes to fish. I've actually shortened the list to include only those with the least amount of fat per ounce. There should be enough choices here to satisfy your needs, yet if you have a yen for a particular fish, look it up in a calorie book. It will probably have more calories per ounce than those listed here, but that simply means you will eat a slightly smaller amount of it. An example is shrimp with 30 calories per ounce. If you would like to have 6 ounces of shrimp (180 calories) for dinner, I'm sure you can make it fit in.

If the fish is purchased fresh, you will need to know the weight of the portion you will be eating in order to calculate the calories. In the case of fish and seafood, I've given you the calorie count per ounce, raw, to make it easy to calculate. If you buy frozen fish, which has nutritional labeling, you can read the number of ounces and the calories directly from the label.

See also "Tuna, Canned" as a separate category in this chapter.

Fish and Seafood (22 calories per ounce)

Cod, Atlantic and Pacific
Crayfish
Monkfish
Pollock, walleye
Pout, ocean
Roughy, orange

Fish and Seafood (26 calories per ounce)

Bass, striped
Catfish, channel, wild
Cisco
Crab, Alaska king
Crab, blue
Crab, Dungeness
Crab, queen
Cusk
Dolphinfish
Flatfish (flounder and sole species)
Grouper, mixed species
Haddock
Ling
Lingcod
Lobster, northern
Ocean perch, Atlantic
Perch, mixed species
Pike, northern
Pike, walleye
Pollock, Atlantic
Rockfish, Pacific, mixed species

Sea bass, mixed species
Sucker, white
Sunfish, pumpkin seed
Tilefish
Turbot, European
Whiting, mixed species
Wolffish, Atlantic

Frozen Meals

This could very well be the best category for a busy person. You simply pop the meal in the microwave and in a few minutes it is ready. I've selected a relatively small number from those available in the supermarket. The selection was based on a careful evaluation of such values as the protein content, the fat content, and the total calories. Remember, these aren't the only frozen foods you may eat, but these are the ones I recommend. As long as you count the total calories and keep track of them, the test will be valid. For maximum hunger control while doing the test, follow my preferences. I've investigated the nutritional content of the most well-known brands. In most cases I had the cooperation of the manufacturers. Bear in mind that the calories provided below are for the entire meal.

HEALTHY CHOICE

Category	Product Label	Calories
Entrée	Swedish Meatballs	280
Entrée	Breaded Chicken Breast Strips	270
Entrée	Chicken & Vegetables Marsala	240
Entrée	Chicken Fettucini Alfredo	280
Entrée	Fiesta Chicken Fajitas	260
Entrée	Grilled Chicken Sonoma	230
Entrée	Grilled Chicken w/Mashed Potatoes	170

Entrée	Homestyle Chicken and Pasta	270
Entrée	Country Roast Turkey w/Mushrooms	230
Meal	Beef & Peppers Cantonese	280
Meal	Traditional Beef Tips	260
Meal	Chicken Broccoli Alfredo	300
Meal	Chicken Cantonese	280
Meal	Chicken Dijon	270
Meal	Roasted Chicken	230
Meal	Southwestern Grilled Chicken	260
Meal	Country Inn Roast Turkey	250
Meal	Traditional Breast of Turkey	290
Bowl Creations	Roasted Potatoes with Ham	200

STOUFFER'S LEAN CUISINE ENTRÉES

Category	Product Label	Calories
American Favorites	Baked Chicken	230
American Favorites	Salisbury Steak	280
Café Classics	Chicken a l'Orange	260
Café Classics	Chicken and Vegetables	270
Café Classics	Chicken in Peanut Sauce	290
Café Classics	Glazed Chicken	240
Café Classics	Herb Roasted Chicken	250
Entrée	Cheese Cannelloni	230
Entrée	Chicken Fettucini	300
Entrée	Homestyle Turkey	230
Hearty Portions	Salisbury Steak	380
Hearty Portions	Grilled Chicken and Penne Pasta	380
Hearty Portions	Oriental Glazed Chicken	350
Hearty Portions	Roasted Chicken with Mushrooms	340

WEIGHT WATCHERS

Product Label	Calories
Chicken Fettucini	300
Slow-Roasted Turkey Breast	220
Chicken Carbonara	300
Penne Pollo	290
Pepper Steak	240
Traditional Lasagna with Meat Sauce	300
Grilled Salisbury Steak and Gravy	290

Fruit, Canned

This is a little easier than fresh since the weights are specified and there is no debris.

	Calories per Ounce
Apple sauce, unsweetened	13
Apricots, water pack	8
Cherries, sweet, water pack	14
Grapefruit, sections, canned	11
Peaches, water pack	7
Pears, water pack	9
Pineapple, water pack	10
Tangerines (mandarin oranges)	11

Fruit, Fresh

If you must have fresh fruit, stick to fruits with lower calories, which means those with the least carbohydrate. It is difficult to calculate the exact calories with fruit, because in many cases you don't eat the entire fruit (the apple core, pits, seeds, etc.). There is also a lot of variation in the calorie count of fruits from different regions.

California grapefruit can have a lot more calories than the Florida variety. How would you calculate the amount of grapefruit you ate? It's difficult. Try to postpone the fresh fruit till after the test.

Fruit, Frozen

Frozen fruit may be regarded similarly to fresh. There is the advantage that because it is packaged, the weight of the contents and the calorie count are specified on the label, and there is generally no debris to subtract. Stay with the lower-calorie varieties, the unsweetened ones. Here are a few:

	Calories per Ounce
Apples	15
Blueberries	16
Boysenberries	15
Cherries	14
Melon balls	11
Strawberries	11

Gelatin Desserts

If you must have dessert, these are probably the best choices. Both Jell-O and Royal have sugar-free varieties. If you make them according to the directions, a ½ cup serving has 10 calories. Jell-O also has ready-to-eat refrigerated portions with 10 calories per little cup.

Grains

You should forgo grains during the test because they are too high in carbohydrate. If you must have them, try to count the calories accurately.

Ketchup

Use a small amount but count it—15 calories per tablespoonful.

Mustard

Mustard is so low in calories that you do not have to count it if you only use a teaspoonful or two.

Nuts and Seeds

Can't you do without these high-fat, high-calorie foods for four weeks?

Pickles

Pickles have always been viewed as the ideal diet snack and they probably deserve the reputation. They are quite low in calories and some of the brands on the shelves indicate "0" calories per serving. Of course that is not quite true; a technicality allows them that license. The FDA permits food producers to round down anything that contains less than 5 calories per serving to zero. You may regard them as a zero-calorie food and not count them in your daily total.

Pork

It may be a surprise that some selected cuts of pork are acceptable. Weigh the separable lean portions only. You can assume an average of 37 calories per ounce:

Pork, fresh, loin, tenderloin, raw
Pork, fresh, loin, sirloin (chops or roasts), boneless, raw
Pork, cured, ham, steak, boneless, extra-lean, unheated

Pork, cured, ham, extra-lean (approximately 4 percent fat), canned, unheated

Pork, cured, ham, extra-lean (approximately 4 percent fat), canned, roasted

Poultry

Chicken and turkey are good choices for this diet. There is surprisingly little difference between the calories per ounce of chicken and turkey and the various cuts, dark or light, of each. Calculate the calories of the raw meat at 32 calories per ounce. Of course no skin or fat should be included.

Soups

Obviously we're speaking of canned or other packaged soups. It would be almost impossible to calculate the calories in homemade soup. Soup is far from my first choice for the test diet. It's essentially a carbohydrate food and sometimes has considerable fat. Soup is in the category of things you may choose to have on infrequent occasions. Just remember to note the calories on the package. Soup made from bouillon cubes or powder is acceptable because it is so low in calories.

Spices, Seasonings, Sauces

In general you may use dry spices to flavor your foods. Some of them have considerable calories per ounce, but what makes them acceptable is the fact that you use so little of them that the amount doesn't even have to be counted. For example, black pepper has 93 calories per ounce, but I doubt that you would ever use enough to give you even 5 calories. In general the seeds that are used as spices, such as celery seed, poppy seed, and caraway seeds, are very high in calories because of their fat content, but if you use them sparingly, you won't have to count them.

Sauces for which only drops are necessary, such as hot sauces, needn't be counted. Some Worcestershire sauces proclaim zero calories, but actually have closer to 5 per teaspoonful. Two teaspoonfuls don't have to be counted.

Tuna, Canned

I have included this as a separate category from "Fish and Seafood" because it is such a popular diet food and it deserves special attention. By now you know that tuna comes packed in water as well as oil, and here I will address only the water-packed variety.

You probably aren't aware of how many different names are used on the labels to describe tuna. "Chunk," "light," "white," "solid," "fillets," "premium," and even others create confusion. Three major brands, Bumble Bee, Starkist, and Chicken of the Sea, all offer satisfactory tunas that contain 60 calories for a 2-ounce serving (¼ cup). That's 30 calories per ounce. Others have more calories. Look for the "60" on the label.

It's not tuna, but a nice variation could be canned Bumble Bee Fancy White Crabmeat with 30 calories per 2-ounce serving.

Vegetables

Vegetables are chosen for their low calorie and low carbohydrate content. Although the selection is somewhat limited, you should be able to manage. If you will be using fresh vegetables, raw or cooked, a food scale is essential so that you can keep an accurate count. It is easier with canned or frozen vegetables, since the package tells you the quantity. Vegetables such as peas may be eaten, but they have a bit more carbohydrate. Regardless of which you choose, if you keep track of the calories, your calculations will come out well.

Vegetables, Raw	Calories per Ounce
Asparagus	8
Beans, kidney	11
Carrots	13
Celery	5
Cucumber, peeled	4
Lettuce, iceberg	4
Lettuce, romaine	5
Mushrooms	9
Onions	11
Peas	24
Radishes	6
Spinach	8
Squash, summer	6
Squash, zucchini	5
Tomatoes	7

Vegetables, Cooked (Drained)	Calories per Ounce
Asparagus	9
Beans, kidney	13
Carrots	13
Cauliflower, cooked	8
Celery	6
Peas	24
Spinach	8
Squash, summer	5
Squash, zucchini	6

Vegetables, Canned (Drained)	Calories per Ounce
Asparagus	7
Beans, snap	5

Carrots	7
Mushrooms	9
Hearts of palm	10
Peas	20

Vegetables, Frozen (Drained)	Calories per Ounce
Asparagus, raw	9
Asparagus, cooked	10
Broccoli, raw	9
Carrots, raw	12
Carrots, cooked	11
Cauliflower, raw	8
Cauliflower, cooked	7
Peas, raw or cooked	23
Squash, zucchini	6

Vinegar

The ordinary varieties have virtually no calories and may be used. The fancier flavored types such as balsamic, which is currently "in," may have from 10 to 40 calories per ounce. Check the label.

Eating Out

The hardest time for keeping track of your calories will be when eating in restaurants. Most restaurants don't supply nutritional information on their foods. By contrast, the most popular fast-food chains do, but they don't generally break down such things as a hamburger sandwich. I've listed the items that are acceptable from some of the fast-food franchises. Remember, if the restaurant posts the calorie count of their super-duper hamburger sandwich, their numbers include the bun, the tomato, the mustard, and everything else. If you eat only the meat and the lettuce, you will have to estimate the calories. Here is where some of the calorie books can really come in handy. Some of them contain data for popular restaurants. Don't neglect keeping track of your calories when you're away from home.

Fast Food

There aren't too many choices in this category. Most fast food is too high in fat or too low in protein. To give you an idea, of the popular hamburgers, Burger King and McDonald's regular hamburgers are listed at 320 calories. Wendy's lists their ¼ pound single burger at 360 with nothing on it, 420 with everything, but the meat patty alone is 200. Its fat content is about 7 percent, a bit high for my kind of diet. Here are some acceptable items:

KFC

Category	Item	Calories per Serving
Original Recipe	Breast with skin removed	129
Tender Roast	Breast with skin removed	169

Note: The information supplied by KFC indicates that the Tender Roast breast meat is a larger portion.

BOSTON MARKET

Item	Calories per Serving
¼ White Meat Chicken without skin or wing	170
Skinless Rotisserie Turkey Breast	170
Chicken Noodle Soup	130
Steamed Vegetables	35
Fruit Salad	70

Vitamins and Minerals

Because of the broad leeway in the choice of foods, it is impossible to be sure that nutritional needs are being met in terms of vitamins and minerals. It is therefore prudent to play it safe by taking daily vitamin-mineral supplements.

There are many satisfactory products on the market. The few suggested below simply represent the type of formula you should be selecting.

Unless you have some specific vitamin deficiency, use the following as a checklist of the minimum amounts the vitamin and mineral supplement should contain:

Vitamin A	5000 I.U.
Vitamin B$_1$ (Thiamine)	1.2 mg.
Vitamin B$_6$ (Pyridoxine)	1.5 mg.
Vitamin B$_{12}$	2.4 mcg.
Vitamin C	90 mg.
Vitamin E	30 I.U.
Vitamin K	80 mg.
Vitamin D	15 mcg.
Vitamin B$_2$ (Riboflavin)	1.3 mg.
Niacin	15 mg.
Folic acid	400 mcg.
Pantothenic acid	5 mg.
Biotin	30 mg.
Choline	550 mg.
Iron	15 mg.
Zinc	15 mg.
Iodine	150 mg.
Selenium	70 mg.
Calcium	1300 mg.
Phosphorus	1250 mg.
Magnesium	410 mg.

If you are already taking a satisfactory combination of vitamins and minerals, there may be no reason to change.

The following are among those that are satisfactory:

Walgreen's
Lederle
Bayer Consumer
Bristol Myers
Therapeutic M
Centrum
One-A-Day Maximum
Theragran-M

It would be a good idea to supplement formulas such as those above with two extra tablets of a calcium/magnesium (500 mg. calcium each) mixture and an extra vitamin C tablet.

Keeping Score

Of course, you're going to try to come as close as possible to 1,000 calories a day. I'm certain that on many days you will deviate by a few calories. There may be other times when you really overdo it. All isn't lost if that happens. What is necessary is for you to know the extent of the variation and to make a note of it. When the twenty-eight days are over, you will have the opportunity to correct the calculations to encompass these variations, but you will need to know exactly what they are. Keep an Excess Calorie Sheet for that purpose.

As an example, if on a particular day your total calories added up to 920, you should make a note on your Excess Calorie Sheet that you were 80 calories under your requirement. You will need to keep a running total of these variations so that at the end of the twenty-eight days you know how many fewer or extra calories you ate during that entire period. I suspect that at the end you will be over rather than under the amount. Remember, don't keep track of the total calories you consumed, only the amounts that were over or under the 1,000.

Here is one more plea for accuracy. There is no point in going through a twenty-eight-day exercise if you won't be able to rely on the outcome. You will lose weight even if you stray somewhat, but we're hoping to get more than weight loss out of these four weeks. During that period you must try to be as precise as possible. After the test is over, if you still have more weight to lose, you may remain on the same diet, but accuracy will not be all that important. A few calories more or less per day may affect the speed of that future weight loss to an extent, but you will have already obtained the information you need.

To repeat, if you stick to packaged foods, it is easier to keep score. Just add up the calories given to you on the package. If you buy "fresh" food, it will require more effort and you will need a food scale, an item that is easily obtainable. Remember to weigh only the portion of the food you will eat. Of course, this means you don't include the bones from meat, what you peel from fruits and vegetables, or what you've left on your plate. If you've weighed a quantity of food and have calculated the calories from the number of ounces but you don't eat it all, you can still calculate the right amount. Weigh the portion you haven't eaten and subtract it. Remember, you're a researcher now performing a very important scientific experiment, and research must be meticulous.

For a sample of daily menus, see Appendix I.

Summing Up

- Appreciate the importance of this exercise. You're collecting valuable information.
- Eat as close to 1,000 calories a day as possible.
- If you deviate from that amount, keep track on an Excess Calorie Sheet of how many more or less calories you've eaten each day.

- For maximum hunger control, try to stick to my food-choice recommendations.
- Follow the diet for exactly twenty-eight days.

13
Evaluating Your Metabolism

Your strict diet is over. Well, maybe not quite. It depends on whether you have reached your proper weight, and in most cases you will not have. Now we're going to find out if your metabolism is as it should be. If it is not, I will tell you how to proceed to lose the rest of your excess weight. If it turns out that your thyroid is working just fine but you still need to lose more weight, I will address that in short order. Let's forget about your diet for a moment and get to the task of calculating your metabolic function index (MFI). I presume it is early in the morning of the day after Day Twenty-eight.

Don't read the rest of this chapter until you've completed the twenty-eight-day diet. If you're impatient and insist on reading on, make sure you reread this when you've completed the diet.

You will be working with the MFI Calculation Form shown on page 161. I won't mind if you slap that page down on a copy machine and copy it and then work from the copy.

MFI Calculation Form

Metabolic Function Index

(1) **Day 1 Date** _____ **Weight (nude)**

(Early morning)

(2) **Day 29 Date** _____ **Weight (nude)**

(Early morning)

(3) **28-day weight loss**

Subtract line (2) from line (1).

(4) **UCML (Uncorrected Caloric Maintenance Level)**

From the UCML Table on page 164.

(5) **EC (Total Excess Calories for the 28 Days)**

From your own list of excess calories for the entire 28 days.

(6) **CCML (Corrected Caloric Maintenance Level)**

See the Excess Calories Table on page 165.

(7) **BBW (Baseline Body Weight)**

See BBW Table on page 166.

(8) **SCML (Standard Caloric Maintenance Level)**

See the proper SCML Table for your sex, age group, and activity level
on pages 168–171. Use the BBW in (7) above to determine your SCML.

(9) **Metabolic Function Index (MFI)**

Divide line (6) by line (8). Move the decimal point
2 digits to the right.

%

Necessary Information

There are a few things you will need to know to make the calculations. One of them is your height in inches. For example: If you're 5 feet 10 inches, you're 70 inches tall.

You will need to decide on your activity level. It will be inactive, moderate, or active. Some examples follow. If you sit at a desk most of the day or you do light housework with no exercise program, you should probably classify yourself as inactive. If you exercise 3 or 4 times a week for about 45 minutes or if your job has you constantly moving and on your feet, you could be in the moderate class. Anything beyond that, such as tennis several times a week, a regular gym workout or jogging, sports activities, etc., probably classifies you as active. I'll elaborate on this just ahead.

When considering such subjects as ideal or normal weight, it is customary to classify individuals by the size of their body "frames." Generally, the classification refers to small, medium, and large frames.

I have found that most people can identify their frame size from their own observations. Anyone who knows you can make an equally authoritative guess. Although it isn't difficult for any of us to judge someone's frame size by our own experience, it is desirable to have some objective standard upon which to rely. One such standard involves taking a measurement across the elbow. The distance between the bony protrusions on the two sides of the elbow are measured. To learn how to do this, go to Appendix D.

The MFI Calculation Form

(1) **Day 1:** You have already filled in the date when you started the diet and your weight on Day 1.

(2) **Day 29:** Now you must fill in your weight on the morning following the twenty-eight-day diet. Next to "Day 29," write in your current weight. If you used your "nude" weight on Day 1,

this should also be the nude weight. The same conditions should prevail in terms of eating, drinking, using the bathroom, etc. If the weight on Day 1 was taken as soon as you emerged from sleep, after going to the bathroom, and before eating or drinking anything, do exactly the same thing now.

(3) **28-Day Weight Loss:** Subtract the second weight from the first weight. Write in the result in the box marked "28-Day Weight Loss."

Calculating the Caloric Maintenance Levels

(4) **UCML (Uncorrected Caloric Maintenance Level):** You're now going to find out your actual caloric maintenance level, which was determined over the twenty-eight-day period. Look on the UCML Table that follows on page 164. UCML stands for uncorrected caloric maintenance level. Find your twenty-eight-day weight loss in the left-hand column. The numbers in the column to the right are the corresponding UCMLs for each weight loss. Write in the UCML on the MFI Calculation Form. This figure represents the number of calories per day it takes to maintain your weight, the number that would have resulted in no weight loss or weight gain over the twenty-eight-day period if you had eaten an average of exactly 1,000 calories per day. Of course, you have kept an Excess Calorie Sheet, and we're going to correct for that next.

(5) **EC (Total Excess Calories for the 28 Days):** If you deviated from the diet on a few occasions and you've kept an Excess Calorie Sheet, total the number of excess calories you consumed for the entire twenty-eight days. If the number is less than 1,400 you may ignore it, but if it is over, mark it in the "EC" box.

(6) **CCML (Corrected Caloric Maintenance Level):** Consult the Excess Calories Table. Locate your total weight loss in the left column. Choose the nearest excess-calorie total across the top of

UCML TABLE
Uncorrected Caloric Maintenance Level

28-DAY WEIGHT LOSS IN POUNDS	UCML
1	1125
2	1250
3	1375
4	1500
5	1625
6	1750
7	1875
8	2000
9	2125
10	2250
11	2375
12	2500
13	2625
14	2750
15	2875
16	3000
17	3125
18	3250
19	3375
20	3500
21	3625
22	3750
23	3875
24	4000
25	4125

Example: *If you've lost 5 pounds during the twenty-eight-day diet, your UCML is 1,625 calories.*

the table. Where the two intersect is your CCML (your corrected caloric maintenance level). Write the CCML in the box on the MFI Calculation Form. If your EC was 1,400 or less, it can be ignored, and your CCML will then be the same as your UCML.

EXCESS CALORIES TABLE
Corrected Caloric Maintenance Level

28-day weight loss	EC (Excess Calories)									
	0	1500	2000	2500	3000	3500	4000	4500	5000	5500
1	1125	1179	1196	1214	1232	1250	1268	1286	1304	1321
2	1250	1304	1321	1339	1357	1375	1393	1411	1429	1446
3	1375	1429	1446	1464	1482	1500	1518	1536	1554	1571
4	1500	1554	1571	1589	1607	1625	1643	1661	1679	1696
5	1625	1679	1696	1714	1732	1750	1768	1786	1804	1821
6	1750	1804	1821	1839	1857	1875	1893	1911	1929	1946
7	1875	1929	1946	1964	1982	2000	2018	2036	2054	2071
8	2000	2054	2071	2089	2107	2125	2143	2161	2179	2196
9	2125	2179	2196	2214	2232	2250	2268	2286	2304	2321
10	2250	2304	2321	2339	2357	2375	2393	2411	2429	2446
11	2375	2429	2446	2464	2482	2500	2518	2536	2554	2571
12	2500	2554	2571	2589	2607	2625	2643	2661	2679	2696
13	2625	2679	2696	2714	2732	2750	2768	2786	2804	2821
14	2750	2804	2821	2839	2857	2875	2893	2911	2929	2946
15	2875	2929	2946	2964	2982	3000	3018	3036	3054	3071
16	3000	3054	3071	3089	3107	3125	3143	3161	3179	3196
17	3125	3179	3196	3214	3232	3250	3268	3286	3304	3321
18	3250	3304	3321	3339	3357	3375	3393	3411	3429	3446
19	3375	3429	3446	3464	3482	3500	3518	3536	3554	3571
20	3500	3554	3571	3589	3607	3625	3643	3661	3679	3696
21	3625	3679	3696	3714	3732	3750	3768	3786	3804	3821
22	3750	3804	3821	3839	3857	3875	3893	3911	3929	3946
23	3875	3929	3946	3964	3982	4000	4018	4036	4054	4071
24	4000	4054	4071	4089	4107	4125	4143	4161	4179	4196
25	4125	4179	4196	4214	4232	4250	4268	4286	4304	4321

Example: If your total weight loss was 5 pounds and you ate an excess of 3,400 calories over the 28-day period, your CCML is 1,750.

(7) **BBW (Baseline Body Weight):** You're now going to find out how many calories a day are needed to maintain weight by a "model" person with your same characteristics. You will need to know the baseline body weight (BBW) for a person of your gender, your height, and your frame size. You will find that weight in the BBW Table that follows. Remember that height is expressed in inches. Find your height in the left column and note the weight that corresponds to your frame size in the columns to the right. Write this in the "BBW" box on the MFI Calculation Form.

BBW TABLE
Baseline Body Weight

	MEN				WOMEN		
Height	SMALL FRAME	MEDIUM FRAME	LARGE FRAME	Height	SMALL FRAME	MEDIUM FRAME	LARGE FRAME
62	117	127	136	58	97	106	115
63	120	130	140	59	99	108	117
64	123	133	143	60	101	111	120
65	126	137	147	61	104	114	123
66	129	140	151	62	107	117	126
67	134	145	156	63	110	120	130
68	138	149	160	64	113	123	133
69	142	153	164	65	116	127	137
70	146	157	168	66	119	130	141
71	150	162	173	67	123	134	145
72	154	166	178	68	127	138	149
73	158	171	183	69	131	142	153
74	162	175	188	70	136	147	158
75	167	180	193	71	140	151	162
76	171	184	197	72	144	156	167

Example: Convert your height to inches. If you're a 5-foot-4-inch female, use 64 inches. If you have a medium frame, the BBW is 123.

(8) SCML (Standard Caloric Maintenance Level): There is a group of tables on pages 168–171 labeled standard caloric maintenance level (SCML). These will tell you how many calories would be required to maintain your proper weight if your metabolism were within normal limits. The multiple SCML tables are geared to your sex, your age, and your activity level. There are three activity levels: sedentary (inactive), moderately active, and active. To help you decide which table applies to you, the following examples may be helpful.

Sedentary: You spend most of the day sitting, occasionally walking for a few minutes at a time. You have no exercise program or at best you exercise an hour or so a week. Examples: secretary, taxi driver, typical desk job.

Moderately Active: You're on your feet most of the day and you do considerable walking. You have an exercise program two to three times a week. Examples: store clerk, nurse, physician, appliance repairman, mail carrier. "Moderately active" can also include someone with a sedentary occupation who exercises three to four times a week or participates in something like swimming or tennis three to four times a week.

Active: Laborer, tile-setter, auto mechanic, furniture mover, in other words a job with no sitting and constant movement all day. Also someone with a more sedentary job who puts in at least an hour of heavy exercise like jogging almost every day might just make it into this category.

Go to the SCML table that is specific for your sex, age group, and activity level. There are twelve different tables for women and the same for men. *Be sure you're using the right table for your age, sex, and activity level.* In the left column find the BBW that is closest to the BBW you've just determined. To the right is the SCML value to be recorded in the box on the MFI Calculation Form. This represents the number of calories that would be needed to maintain your weight if you had a normal metabolism.

SCML TABLE FOR WOMEN
Standard Caloric Maintenance Level

SEDENTARY AGE 16-18		MODERATELY ACTIVE AGE 16-18		ACTIVE AGE 16-18	
BBW	SCML	BBW	SCML	BBW	SCML
100	1821	100	2081	100	2601
110	1898	110	2170	110	2712
120	1976	120	2258	120	2823
130	2054	130	2347	130	2934
140	2131	140	2436	140	3045
150	2209	150	2525	150	3156
160	2287	160	2613	160	3267
170	2364	170	2702	170	3377
180	2442	180	2791	180	3488

SEDENTARY AGE 19-30		MODERATELY ACTIVE AGE 19-30		ACTIVE AGE 19-30	
BBW	SCML	BBW	SCML	BBW	SCML
100	1630	100	1863	100	2328
110	1723	110	1970	110	2462
120	1817	120	2077	120	2596
130	1910	130	2183	130	2729
140	2004	140	2290	140	2863
150	2098	150	2397	150	2997
160	2191	160	2504	160	3130
170	2285	170	2611	170	3264
180	2378	180	2718	180	3397

SCML TABLE FOR WOMEN (continued)

SEDENTARY AGE 31-60		MODERATELY ACTIVE AGE 31-60		ACTIVE AGE 31-60	
BBW	SCML	BBW	SCML	BBW	SCML
100	1714	100	1959	100	2449
110	1770	110	2022	110	2528
120	1825	120	2086	120	2607
130	1880	130	2149	130	2686
140	1936	140	2212	140	2765
150	1991	150	2275	150	2844
160	2046	160	2339	160	2923
170	2102	170	2402	170	3003
180	2157	180	2465	180	3082

SEDENTARY AGE over 60		MODERATELY ACTIVE AGE over 60		ACTIVE AGE over 60	
BBW	SCML	BBW	SCML	BBW	SCML
100	1503	100	1717	100	2147
110	1569	110	1794	110	2242
120	1636	120	1870	120	2337
130	1703	130	1946	130	2433
140	1770	140	2023	140	2528
150	1837	150	2099	150	2624
160	1903	160	2175	160	2719
170	1970	170	2252	170	2815
180	2037	180	2328	180	2910

SCML TABLE FOR MEN
Standard Caloric Maintenance Level

SEDENTARY AGE 16-18		MODERATELY ACTIVE AGE 16-18		ACTIVE AGE 16-18	
BBW	SCML	BBW	SCML	BBW	SCML
100	2025	100	2459	100	3182
110	2136	110	2594	110	3357
120	2248	120	2729	120	3532
130	2359	130	2865	130	3707
140	2470	140	3000	140	3882
150	2582	150	3135	150	4057
160	2693	160	3270	160	4232
170	2805	170	3406	170	4407
180	2916	180	3541	180	4582
190	3027	190	3676	190	4757
200	3139	200	3811	200	4932
210	3250	210	3946	210	5107
220	3361	220	4082	220	5282

SEDENTARY AGE 19-30		MODERATELY ACTIVE AGE 19-30		ACTIVE AGE 19-30	
BBW	SCML	BBW	SCML	BBW	SCML
100	1924	100	2337	100	3024
110	2022	110	2455	110	3177
120	2119	120	2573	120	3330
130	2216	130	2691	130	3483
140	2314	140	2809	140	3636
150	2411	150	2928	150	3789
160	2508	160	3046	160	3942
170	2606	170	3164	170	4095
180	2703	180	3282	180	4248
190	2801	190	3401	190	4401
200	2898	200	3519	200	4554
210	2995	210	3637	210	4707
220	3093	220	3755	220	4860

SCML TABLE FOR MEN (continued)

SEDENTARY AGE 31-60		MODERATELY ACTIVE AGE 31-60		ACTIVE AGE 31-60	
BBW	SCML	BBW	SCML	BBW	SCML
100	1969	100	2391	100	3094
110	2043	110	2480	110	3210
120	2116	120	2570	120	3326
130	2190	130	2660	130	3442
140	2264	140	2749	140	3558
150	2338	150	2839	150	3674
160	2412	160	2928	160	3790
170	2486	170	3018	170	3906
180	2559	180	3108	180	4022
190	2633	190	3197	190	4138
200	2707	200	3287	200	4254
210	2781	210	3377	210	4370
220	2855	220	3466	220	4486

SEDENTARY AGE over 60		MODERATELY ACTIVE AGE over 60		ACTIVE AGE over 60	
BBW	SCML	BBW	SCML	BBW	SCML
100	1541	100	1871	100	2421
110	1627	110	1975	110	2556
120	1713	120	2080	120	2691
130	1799	130	2184	130	2826
140	1885	140	2288	140	2961
150	1970	150	2393	150	3096
160	2056	160	2497	160	3231
170	2142	170	2601	170	3366
180	2228	180	2706	180	3501
190	2314	190	2810	190	3636
200	2400	200	2914	200	3771
210	2486	210	3019	210	3906
220	2572	220	3123	220	4041

> **Example:** *If you're a 5-foot-4-inch female with a medium frame, you've determined that your BBW is 123 pounds. If you're age 35 and moderately active, the table lists your SCML as 2,086 calories.*

For more help with determining your activity level, see Appendix E.

(9) Metabolic Function Index (MFI): Now divide the CCML by the SCML. Move the decimal point two digits to the right and round it off to a whole number. This represents your metabolic function index stated as a percentage. Write this in the "MFI" box.

> **Example:** *Divide your CCML, 1,750, by your SCML, 2,086. The result is 0.839. Now move the decimal point two digits to the right (83.9) and round it off to 84. Your MFI is 84 percent.*

Interpretation of the MFI Results

The lower the percentage, the lower is your metabolic rate. There is room for error throughout the test and the calculations, so that a minimal deviation from 100 percent should not be considered as necessarily abnormal. I regard 90 percent as the borderline, and I would consider 90 percent as an indication of very mild hypothyroidism. As the MFI percentage falls lower, the likelihood of hypothyroidism becomes more certain. At 80 percent, I believe we have full-blown hypothyroidism, and some people will have an MFI much lower than that. We will still want to confirm our results with the corroborating tests that follow.

An MFI of 80 percent would represent a female who in order to maintain her weight must eat 400 calories a day less than another female who doesn't have hypothyroidism. I would also expect that the hypothyroid female would have several annoying symptoms not possessed by the normal individual.

In my practice, I've seen patients who have had an MFI as low as 60 percent, and I have had others whose medical histories would have suggested an even lower MFI, but they didn't have the discipline to allow us to perform an accurate test. I don't know what the lower limit of MFI is, but I'm sure it would impress even me.

Let's go over the examples given above. The hypothetical five-foot-four-inch lady who lost five pounds during her twenty-eight-day test diet didn't lose as much as a "normal" person would have lost. Had she eaten during that period the number of calories that would have maintained her weight, she would have had to have eaten 1,750 calories a day. The normal person of her same type would have maintained her weight on 2,086 calories. Our lady needs only 84 percent of the calories of that normal person. Her 84 percent classifies her as hypothyroid. Recognize that there is room for error in the entire process. A value of 90 percent is a questionable indicator of hypothyroidism. It is a borderline case in which I have to make an intelligent decision, and I can't do that without considering all of her information. In my opinion, the 84 percent is reason enough to treat her.

The MFI should give you a clear-cut look at how you handle calories in the real world. It isn't based on mysterious laboratory tests done behind closed doors by machines that are as subject to error as the individuals who operate them. I feel that the results of the MFI are almost irrefutable. Yes, it is true that you could have weighed yourself incorrectly or you may have used an inaccurate scale. You could have been mistaken as to your height. You might have suppressed remembering your true age, and your arithmetic could be shameful. But if you do your work carefully, the result is valid. It represents a study done by a real human being, on a real human being, in the real world, with real food. The resulting weight loss is real. If it turns out that you need 25 percent less food in order to maintain your weight than someone else does who is much like you, who would argue that there isn't something different about your metabolism?

Let's now see if another test corroborates what we've learned about you. Look at the Daily Temperature Chart below. In Chapter 11 you were asked to write in your temperature on Day 1.

DAILY TEMPERATURE CHART

Date	Temperature
1	_____
2	_____
3	_____
4	_____
5	_____
6	_____
7	_____
8	_____
9	_____
10	_____
11	_____
12	_____
13	_____
14	_____
15	_____
16	_____
17	_____
18	_____
19	_____
20	_____
21	_____
22	_____
23	_____
24	_____
25	_____
26	_____
27	_____
28	_____
Total	_____

A. Total of Temperature Column _____

B. Total Number of Readings _____

C. Average Daily Temperature _____
   Divide A by B

D. **Temperature Difference**

If you've followed instructions, there should be from 15 to 28 temperature readings recorded on the chart. I'm going to ask you to add up all the temperature readings and put the total on the line labeled "Total of Temperature Column." You may want to use a calculator for that and the next step. Now count the number of readings. It should be 15 or more. Place that number on the line labeled "Total Number of Readings." Now divide the total of the temperature readings by the number of readings. This will give you the average daily temperature, which you should place on that line. If the average daily temperature (ADT) is greater than 98.6 degrees, subtract 98.6 from the ADT and place it in the box labeled "Temperature Difference," putting a plus sign (+) in front of it. If the average daily temperature (ADT) is less than 98.6, subtract the ADT from 98.6 and place it in the box labeled "Temperature Difference" and put a minus sign (–) in front of it.

> **Example:** *You've added up 18 temperature readings and they total 1742.4. Divide by 18. The ADT is 96.8. Subtract 96.8 from 98.6. The result is a temperature difference of –1.8.*

For an interpretation of this, I will go back to Dr. Broda Barnes, who had great confidence in this test. In his experience he found that a temperature from one to three degrees below normal was indicative of hypothyroidism. Obviously, the lower the temperature the more certain and perhaps the more severe is the hypothyroidism. Therefore, a temperature difference of –1 is suspicious. A difference of –2 or even –3 definitely points in the direction of hypothyroidism. This is information that you will want to present to your doctor when the time comes.

Incidentally, if you have positive numbers for the temperature difference, this should also be investigated. Such a constant fever isn't normal either, but it indicates an entirely different problem, possibly infection. It might also suggest an overabundance of thyroid hormone, which could mean hyperthyroidism. In any case, this constant fever should be reported to your doctor.

Now we will go on to an entirely different kind of test to corroborate our findings in the MFI test. The signs and symptoms of hypothyroidism described earlier are quite helpful in making the diagnosis. In fact the more of these that are present, the more certain the diagnosis. Even though I've seen cases where only two or three signs or symptoms were present, I don't think I've ever seen a case where more than four or five were present and the patient didn't have hypothyroidism. I've adapted tests done by other researchers to fit the needs of the layman who wants to investigate whether his own symptoms suggest hypothyroidism.

The test we will do is essentially taken from the Billewicz index, a well-regarded method of evaluating hypothyroidism without laboratory tests. This should serve the reader well in providing additional corroborating evidence to be presented to the physician.

The Signs and Symptoms Index Form follows on page 179. You're asked to decide yes or no as to how each of them applies to you. Your answers must be definite. There is no "maybe" answer. So choose what is more probable, yes or no. Instead of putting down a check mark, you're asked to circle the number under either "Yes" or "No." You must circle one or the other for each of the items. Don't skip any. The numbers assigned to each symptom are a method of assigning a relative importance to each of them. Note that a yes or no answer for the same symptom may not have the same value. This was a well-conceived bit of research by those who developed the questionnaire.

Some of these will be hard or impossible for you to evaluate on your own. You will need help. With some you may wish to ask the opinion of someone else who knows you. Let's try to get accurate answers. The following section will give you some help with determining whether to put down a yes or no for the individual items.

Diminished Sweating: You can decide this for yourself. I've had many patients who have told me, "I never perspire." Whether that is exactly true or not, it is sufficient that they think that they perspire less than they should, less than the average person. For yes, circle the 6, for no, circle the 2.

Dry Skin: This one is easy. You don't have to ask anyone else. You should have an impression. Circle 3 for yes, circle 6 for no.

Cold Intolerance: Not everyone with hypothyroidism feels cold, but some people do. Are you frequently cold? Are you the one who needs a sweater when everyone else seems comfortable? Circle 4 for yes, circle 5 for no.

Weight Increase: Here I've taken license with the original intent of the authors of the study. If you've had an unexpected, unexplained weight gain that didn't seem to be related to an increase in your intake of food, answer yes. If you feel that you're overweight and it isn't justified by the amount you eat, answer yes. Circle the 1 in the proper column.

Constipation: Another easy one. You feel either that you are or that you are not. Circle 2 for yes, 1 for no.

Hoarseness:* This is one where you may ask the opinions of those around you. Often we don't know what our own voice sounds like. Have you heard a tape recording of your voice? If there has been a change in the character of your voice, you may not be aware of it. Circle 5 for yes, 6 for no.

Numbness: I have translated this from the medical word, paresthesia, which also might include tingling or a prickly feeling. It could be anywhere on the body, as long as it is bothersome and has no other explanation. Circle 5 for yes, 4 for no.

Deafness:* I don't mean total deafness. This is anything that leads you to believe you don't hear as well as you should. You may want to ask the opinions of others. Circle 2 for yes, 0 for no.

Slow Movements:* Here is where friends and family can be of help. The question is, Do you seem to move more slowly than most people? It isn't simply whether you're a couch potato or not, or someone who would rather read or watch TV than do physical things. It goes beyond that. Are your movements actually slower than those of others? Think about it. We all know people who do everything quickly and have jerky movements. This is the opposite. There are those who move at the proverbial snail's pace. This is an important one. Try to get an accurate answer. Circle 11 for yes, 3 for no.

Coarse Skin:* You should be able to answer this very quickly. Circle 7 under either yes or no.

Cold Skin:* You can't determine the temperature of your own skin. Ask others if you usually have cold skin. Circle 3 for yes, or 2 for no.

Puffiness Around Eyes: Again, your opinion along with assistance from others should help you come up with the answer. Circle 4 for yes, 6 for no.

Pulse Rate: Do you know how to take your own pulse? You should. It is very useful. Learn how. For the present, find someone who seems to know what they are doing and let him do it, and while you're at it, get him to teach you how. Sit for a few minutes and then count the number of heartbeats for a full minute (sixty seconds). If it is 66 or less, circle the 4 for yes, otherwise circle the 4 for no.

Calculating Your Signs and Symptoms Index

Use the Signs and Symptoms Index Form that follows.

The Signs and Symptoms Index Form

Circle the number under "**Yes**" or "**No**" that best describes you. You may want to ask the opinion of others for the four items with asterisks (*). See explanation of signs and symptoms that precedes this form (pages 176–78).

	YES	NO
Diminished Sweating	6	2
Dry Skin	3	6
Cold Intolerance	4	5
Weight Increase	1	1
Constipation	2	1
Hoarseness*	5	6
Numbness	5	4
Deafness*	2	0
Slow Movements*	11	3
Coarse Skin	7	7
Cold Skin*	3	2
Puffiness Around Eyes	4	6
Pulse Rate	4	4
Total of Each Column	____	____
Index Score *(Subtract Column 2 from Column 1)*	_____	

Add up all the circled numbers in the "Yes" column and put the total below. Add up all the circled numbers in the "No" column and put the total below.

Subtract the total of the "No" column from the total of the "Yes" column. That is your index score.

A score of 25 or greater strongly suggests hypothyroidism. A score of 20 to 24 is suspicious. A score below that doesn't rule out hypothyroidism. It is still quite possible. The higher scores do tend to confirm a low MFI index.

A comment on the test seems to be in order. The test was designed by researchers and was intended to be used by doctors for evaluating patients. It wasn't intended for the layman to test himself. Certainly, testing oneself does introduce a new possibility of subjective error. Still, I'm not sure that a doctor is better than your best friend at evaluating your hoarseness or your slow movements.

I have purposely omitted one very important sign that the researchers included: the sluggishness of the ankle jerk. If you will recall, I spoke earlier about the Achilles reflex test, a test I particularly liked. The researchers who developed the symptoms test were drawing on this same phenomenon. They wanted the doctor to evaluate the movement of the ankle after the tendon had been tapped with a medical hammer. This takes some experience, both to give the tap as well as to evaluate the result. We don't want any broken bones when someone enthusiastically applies a sledgehammer to the ankle. But, as a result of the omission, the test isn't exactly as it was intended. A yes to the ankle-jerk test would have added a significant 15 points, whereas a normal reflex would have subtracted only 6. This could tend to throw the interpretation values I've given you off a bit. The error would be in the direction of underestimating who has hypothyroidism. I'm going to stick to my guns. I think as the test has been given to you, it should prove quite useful.

Putting the Tests into Perspective

We have performed the principal test and two corroborating tests. Remember that I've applied these very principles in my own practice over many years on thousands and thousands of patients. They've served me and my patients well. I really want to share this information. I don't believe that such a systematic approach to self-help in discovering hypothyroidism has ever been presented to the public.

Could some find fault with the theory, the methods, and the interpretation? Of course. You can find fault with anything. Is it perfect? Obviously not. What in medicine or in any other discipline is perfect? This is, however, a serious attempt to fill a gap I believe exists. More importantly, I believe it can help a sizable number of our population.

Let's go on to how you may use the information you've obtained.

Summing Up

- Calculating the results of the MFI test gives the reader a clear-cut view of whether his or her thyroid function is normal.
- An additional corroborating test measures body temperature for evaluation as a sign of hypothyroidism.
- A test based on a questionnaire of symptoms provides further corroboration.

14
Weight Loss Without Guesswork

This chapter is full of assumptions.

I will assume that you've done a fine job of conducting the MFI test and that you're now ready to put the results to good use. You've followed the instructions meticulously and have arrived at a good estimate of how your thyroid functions. There are various possible outcomes of your testing. You may have learned that you burn up calories every bit as efficiently as the next person, and as a consequence there is no reason why any sensible low-calorie diet would not work for you.

Or you may have learned that you don't burn calories properly. You haven't lost the pounds that were expected on a 1,000-calorie diet. Worse, you may have lost so little that considerable hypothyroidism is indicated. In any case, you're being rewarded for your effort with valuable information. The solution to the problem isn't yet obvious, but you have the information that can help you find that solution. Let's look at the possibilities.

Your Metabolism Is Normal and You Have Weight to Lose

Here is one of those assumptions. Your MFI test gave you a value of 96 percent. Though that is a few points below 100 percent, the theoretical normal, this isn't low enough to suggest a thyroid problem. There is too much room for variation in the different aspects of the test to call 96 percent hypothyroidism. Bear in mind that it is still possible. You may have deviated from procedure enough that 96 percent should really have been, say, 89 percent, in which case we would suspect mild hypothyroidism or what the literature commonly calls subclinical hypothyroidism.

At anything above 90 percent, I would make the assumption that I didn't have hypothyroidism and get to work losing weight with a sensible diet. The diet you followed during the 28-day test is a sensible diet and, what's more, I know it works. So why not get busy and just do it?

Should you handle the diet differently as your weight-loss diet than you did as your test diet? Somewhat. You don't have to be as scrupulously exact as I asked you to be during the test. We're no longer gathering information. The 1,000-calorie diet should continue to result in weight loss and at about the same rate it did during the test. If you lost ten pounds during the test, you will probably lose another ten in the next four weeks. You certainly don't have to keep an Excess Calorie Sheet. A few more calories a day or a few less will probably not be noticed.

Can you increase the number of calories per day? The answer is yes, but you will have to pay the price, a slower rate of weight loss. I find that motivated patients generally tolerate a 1,000-calorie diet quite well. In my own practice, I actually use an 800-calorie diet, but I watch my patients very carefully. This will have to be a decision for your own doctor to make. I would recommend that you don't pressure your doctor to approve a lesser number of calories than he seems comfortable with, and I certainly don't recommend that you go against your doctor's orders.

Bear in mind that each 125-calorie-per-day addition to your

diet is expected to result in 1 pound less of weight loss for the four-week period. Thus, if you change to a 1,250-calorie diet, you will be expected to lose 2 pounds less than with a 1,000-calorie diet.

You may ask, "Why not eat a few hundred more calories per day and be more comfortable even though you lose a little slower?" The answer is that I'm not sure you will be more comfortable. It has never seemed to me that patients enjoyed a 1,200-calorie diet any more than they did an 800-calorie diet. Let's face it. Dieting isn't fun. Its justification is the reward at the end. That vision of a slim body is a powerful motivator. But fun it is not. The impression that we're asked to get from watching television commercials for weight-loss products suggests that the process of losing weight is one of the great joys of life. Let's get rid of those unrealistic expectations. The joy is in the result, not in the process.

There is another reason for fewer calories and faster weight loss. It is my impression, gleaned from those thousands of patients, that the longer losing weight takes, the less likely it is to be successful. Success is a two-pronged affair. It should be noted here that I define the first stage of success as reaching the particular goal weight that was set in the beginning. The final step in success is maintaining that weight for a lifetime.

I have noted that patients who frequently falter along the way are less likely to reach their goal weights. The opposite is certainly true. The patient who exhibits fanaticism and who never deviates virtually always achieves the goal, and of course it is done in record time. That kind of patient completes that important first step and is eager to do what is necessary to maintain that new figure for a lifetime.

If you choose to go much above 1,000 calories per day, I believe you will lower your odds of success. I must tell you that I'm not a gambler by nature. I like the odds to be on my side, not on the side of the "house." I think you slant the odds in your favor when you follow my 1,000-calorie diet.

In spite of what I've just said about my preference for 1,000 calories per day, I can at least show you what to expect in the way of weight loss if you go above 1,000 per day. The chart that follows is based upon a twenty-eight-day period. You may wonder why I consistently gravitate to exactly four weeks. It is because of the extreme variability of weight loss when viewed over a shorter period. My own medical practice is geared to reevaluation every four weeks, even though I'm seeing the patient more frequently than that. I find that weight comparisons over four weeks are reliable. The table that follows on page 186 shows you how much weight loss to expect in a four-week period based upon your corrected caloric maintenance level, which you learned from the MFI test. I told you that the information would prove valuable to you, and this is but one example of that. In the table, find your CCML (corrected caloric maintenance level) in the left column that matches your CCML on Line (6) on your MFI Calculation Form (page 161). Across the top of the table are the various daily calorie counts for the diet you are or will be following. Where the two intersect is the expected twenty-eight-day weight loss. If you've done the MFI test diligently, you will be surprised how accurate a predictor of weight loss this is.

Here is another way you can keep the odds in your favor. Every diet book tells you to see your doctor before you start a diet. I generally have the impression that this advice is given without much conviction that it's really necessary or that the reader will follow it. I really believe you should see your doctor, not just at the beginning, but also during the course of the diet. I will give you my reasons.

We're looking for success, and I've defined success as permanently achieving a proper weight. Again, I will refer to the odds. It is my impression that my patients have a greater chance for success in achieving the weight objective with the help of my overseeing the process than do those who try to do it on their own. They are certainly more successful than those who try those kooky schemes that are advertised so widely. I would like to think this success stems entirely from my superior knowledge of dieting methods, but unfortunately I cannot give myself that much

TABLE OF EXPECTED WEIGHT LOSS
Pounds Lost in 28 Days on Various Calorie Diets

CCML	Daily Calorie Count of Diet				
	1000	1200	1400	1600	1800
1000	0	-1.6	-3.2	-4.8	-6.4
1100	0.8	-0.8	-2.4	-4	-5.6
1200	1.6	0	-1.6	-3.2	-4.8
1300	2.4	0.8	-0.8	-2.4	-4
1400	3.2	1.6	0	-1.6	-3.2
1500	4	2.4	0.8	-0.8	-2.4
1600	4.8	3.2	1.6	0	-1.6
1700	5.6	4	2.4	0.8	-0.8
1800	6.4	4.8	3.2	1.6	0
1900	7.2	5.6	4	2.4	0.8
2000	8	6.4	4.8	3.2	1.6
2100	8.8	7.2	5.6	4	2.4
2200	9.6	8	6.4	4.8	3.2
2300	10.4	8.8	7.2	5.6	4
2400	11.2	9.6	8	6.4	4.8
2500	12	10.4	8.8	7.2	5.6
2600	12.8	11.2	9.6	8	6.4
2700	13.6	12	10.4	8.8	7.2
2800	14.4	12.8	11.2	9.6	8
2900	15.2	13.6	12	10.4	8.8
3000	16	14.4	12.8	11.2	9.6
3100	16.8	15.2	13.6	12	10.4
3200	17.6	16	14.4	12.8	11.2
3300	18.4	16.8	15.2	13.6	12
3400	19.2	17.6	16	14.4	12.8
3500	20	18.4	16.8	15.2	13.6

Note: Minus values indicate a weight gain.

credit. The phenomenon of the patient having to make regular visits to my office, to confront my staff, to face me directly on a regular basis, is probably as responsible for their success as is the actual method used. That is one reason, a very good reason, why you should diet under the auspices of your doctor. In case I didn't make the reason clear enough, I will state it succinctly: *Conducting your diet with your doctor's help will increase your chances for success.*

Another reason for working with your doctor is safety. You should be examined before you embark on a diet. For one thing, it is a good excuse to have a physical. Who knows what demons are lurking inside you, unrelated to diet! He will undoubtedly do lab work first, and an electrocardiogram is always advisable. Play it safe. Let's do this the right way.

It's probably a good idea to reread Chapter 11 before you go on with the diet. The advice given for my preferences in the various lists and text are still applicable. Get started. Let's get that weight off.

Bear in mind that I'm speaking of you, the reader, and this section deals with the reader who doesn't have a thyroid problem impeding weight loss. For those who do have an abnormal MFI test result, the road to success with the doctor could be a rockier one.

Your MFI Test Is Abnormal

Suppose your test result is 90 percent or lower. Depending on how low it is, losing weight could turn out to be a real burden. You may be in a category of patients I see all too often. These are people who suspect something is wrong, and often have been told there is nothing wrong. If your result is 80 percent or lower, it would be difficult, taking all the factors into consideration, to conclude that there is nothing wrong. A value of 80 percent could represent someone who cannot maintain her weight on a diet of about 1,600 calories a day when she should be maintaining at the 2,000-calorie level. I would also be willing to bet that someone with that score would also have several of the symptoms of hypothyroidism I've previously covered. You will probably have body temperature at least one degree below "normal," and there is a good chance that you complain of always feeling tired. The work is cut out for you. A doctor must be found, one who will listen, and an effort must be made to correct the problem.

Your first choice should be your family doctor or your "primary care physician," as they are now called. Make the appointment and be prepared for resistance. Your job is to let him know about your symptoms of hypothyroidism. You should previously have copied and filled out the "letter to your doctor" that follows. You must get across the information that you've just completed a test where you ate 1,000 calories per day for four weeks and you lost only a certain number of pounds. Tell him that you followed exact instructions to determine how many pounds would have been lost by a "normal" person like you and that your percentage of that amount was low enough to indicate you weren't normal.

The form letter that follows on page 189 is a summary of the tests you've performed. It is presented in a simplified manner and is intended to supply information about you to your doctor. Fill in the blanks. Make a photocopy of it if you like. The information that is asked for is on your MFI Calculation Form.

Your 28-day weight loss goes in blank (3).
Your daily caloric maintenance level (CCML) goes in blank (4).
The theoretical caloric maintenance level (SCML) goes in blank (5).
Your percentage of normal (MFI) goes in blank (6).
Your average daily temperature, which goes in blank (7), is on your Daily Temperature Chart in Chapter 13.
Your signs and symptoms score is on the Signs and Symptoms Index Form (also in Chapter 13).

My guess is that your doctor will say this is interesting and that the next step is to test your thyroid. You already know my feelings on that subject, but it would be prudent not to object, although you might point out that you've just read a book in which

---

Date _____

Dear Dr. _____

I have just completed a home test specified in a book by Dr. Sanford Siegal titled *Is Your Thyroid Making You Fat?* The test compares how I burn calories as compared to a normal individual with my same characteristics. I have followed a 1,000-calorie-per-day diet for twenty-eight days and have carefully recorded my weight change during that time.

Here are the results:

I lost _____ pounds over the 28-day period.
          (3)

My daily caloric maintenance level was calculated to be _____ calories.
                                                                      (4)

Theoretically, a person like me should maintain weight at _____ calories.
                                                                     (5)

My caloric maintenance level is _____ percent of that of a normal person.
                                           (6)

Additionally, my daily body temperature averages _____° F.
                                                           (7)

I answered questions regarding my symptoms of hypothyroidism and received a score of _____. Dr. Siegal has suggested that a score of 25 or greater is suspicious of hypothyroidism.

I hope this information will prove helpful.

Sincerely,

_____

---

the author casts doubt on the value of such testing. Except that you may have to pay for the testing, there is no reason not to have it done. For one thing, your TSH test may come back elevated and your doctor will then accept the fact that you're hypothyroid. This is the path of least resistance. You will still have one more hurdle, but we will get to that soon enough.

This is neither the best-case scenario nor the worst. The best would be if your physician told you that he was aware that thyroid tests are questionable, that he was aware of my book and was pretty much in agreement, and that since you had all the earmarks of hypothyroidism, including a high cholesterol, he was going to give you a cautious try on thyroid hormone treatment. Don't expect that to happen. Instead, hope he will just listen.

There is more ammunition you can use. Chapter 15 in this book is written just for him. It takes into account that your doctor is a busy man, so I've tried to summarize the whole issue into as few words as possible. You might just get lucky. He might just read it.

There is even more. Virtually everyone is into the Internet these days. Tell him that I have a Web site (drsiegal.com) that will give him even more information. If he will contact the site, I will send him more information that may sway his thinking. Of course the information will not be about you personally, but it will summarize the concepts contained in my book. There is even another alternative. My Web site will allow you to request that I send him the information, and he will know you made the request.

Suppose all fails. Your doctor is unmoved. He says there is nothing wrong with your thyroid and tells you to follow this or that diet and quit worrying. You will then have a decision to make. If his arguments seem stronger than mine, the decision should not be difficult. If you feel you haven't had a fair hearing, you have other choices. You may even ask for his cooperation in this. Second opinions among doctors are a standard procedure. He should not even mind recommending a colleague for that opinion. A few doctors are insecure enough that they regard someone's seeking a second opinion as a threat of some sort or at least a questioning of their competence. Let's hope your doctor isn't one of those.

You may run into the same problem with other doctors. My own Web site may be of help. I've started collecting the names of physicians around the country who have taken an interest in my findings and who, to varying degrees, have observed what I have and are willing to keep an open mind when it comes to thyroid problems. I expect the list to grow, and I would gladly share names of doctors in your area with you. Again, my Web site will be your source for this information. Look for it at:

www.drsiegal.com.

The second hurdle I spoke of has to do with the choice of thyroid hormone to treat your problem. You've been told repeatedly that the vast majority of doctors treat hypothyroidism with synthetic thyroid, also known as levothyroxine or thyroxine or T4. You also know that synthetic isn't my choice. I consistently get better results by prescribing natural thyroid, otherwise known as Thyroid U.S.P. or desiccated thyroid, or sometimes Armour. Again, I will make the point that synthetic thyroid works for many patients. I just find that natural thyroid works better. Ideally, I would like to see your hypothyroidism treated with natural thyroid. Since it is a recognized and accepted medication available in all pharmacies, you may have less of a problem getting that point across than the previous one. My Web site (and others) may be able to help you find a doctor who will prescribe natural thyroid.

Let's now adopt a positive outlook. Your doctor accepts that you're hypothyroid and has prescribed one of the varieties of thyroid hormone. He should schedule frequent visits to assess the value of the medication you're taking. I believe that for the first year you should be reevaluated each month for the proper dosage. Since I don't consider the laboratory a suitable indicator for proper dosage, the determination becomes somewhat of an art. (Medicine in general has sometimes been characterized as an art rather than a science.) Still, there are objective signs, and I'm sure that your physician will monitor them. Your blood-cholesterol reading could help. Of course it will also be influenced by your diet. Your temperature will tell him something. Your blood pressure and your pulse rate contribute. Mostly the information that you report will tell the story. Nothing tells me more than the patient reporting, "I no longer have that terrible tired feeling."

As for your weight-loss diet, there is no reason why it should be very different from what was spoken of in the previous section, the one dealing with the reader who doesn't have a thyroid problem. If you're treated correctly, you too will not have a thyroid problem, or at least it will be corrected by supplying the right hormones. Your weight loss in this corrected condition should be the same as for a "normal" person.

If the assumption is that you've suspected your metabolism wasn't normal and you have been frustrated in efforts to confirm that suspicion, the MFI test should go a long way toward ending that frustration. Do the test, present your findings, and get on with feeling better. It is worth the effort.

Getting the Job Done

Staying with a diet is a task that requires as much thought and planning as any other major undertaking in your life. I happen to think that achieving a normal weight should be a high-priority item on your agenda. I'm often shocked at how casually some people regard this matter. They may pay lip service to how badly they want to lose weight, but often their subsequent behavior makes that concern somewhat suspect.

I have seen overachievers whose lives are organized to the hilt conduct their weight-losing effort in a shamefully slipshod manner. What is required, as with any other task worth doing, is planning. Plan each day in advance. What will you eat that day? Where will it come from? What forces could intervene to sidetrack your efforts? How will you counter those problems?

The support of others—a spouse, a friend, a parent—can be helpful, but don't count on it. I don't know how many times I have been told, "I don't get any support from my . . ." It would be nice if those who profess to love us would do what they could to make the job easier, but help is not always there, and an exploration of the psychological overtones of why it is not is beyond the scope of this book.

"My husband likes to go out and eat good meals on the weekends and I can't just sit there and eat lettuce."

"Here I am trying my best to get healthy and she makes these

fantastic meals. I don't know if she tries to make them more en-
ticing when I'm dieting or if they just seem that way."

Of course, such actions on the part of those who purport to
love us provide a very convenient excuse for why we can't succeed.
In the end, you have to stand on your own two feet and get the
job done. If you count on support, it may not be there.

I'm reminded of an incident where the lack of support was not
very subtle. Mariola came to me weighing 212, a bit much for her
five-foot-four-inch small frame. She was doing fabulously well.
She had mentioned that her husband did not want her to get
down as low as I had suggested, but I sort of ignored that hint.
She had reached 180 when I received a phone call from him. "I
don't want her to lose any more weight." Without asking why, I
tried to explain why she should. He cut me off, and this time his
anger was apparent. "No more," he said emphatically. I knew it
would be hard for him to understand this, but I had to tell him.
"Mr. ———, I'm really not permitted to discuss your wife's medical treatment with you without her permission. Even though you
are her husband, the rules say that I may not talk to you about
her. I'm really very sorry, but . . ." Again he wasn't interested in
my explanation. His voice was now quite loud. "If she loses any
more weight, I'll be out there to get you." He hung up.

Thank goodness he never did appear, principally I suppose because she never reappeared. Obviously, he used other means to
solve his problem.

Your husband, your wife, your boyfriend, girlfriend, or who-
ever may not be as assertive as Mariola's husband, so don't be
shocked if you are not receiving the support you believe you deserve. Like many other tasks in life, losing weight is a lonely one.

Medication for Weight Loss

The subject of medications for suppressing hunger during a
weight-loss diet has become rather controversial as a result of the
unfortunate phen-fen interlude. You will recall that a combina-

tion of two medications, both approved but not sanctioned as a combination by the Food and Drug Administration, was being passed out rather indiscriminately by a variety of opportunistic health-care providers with resultant harm to a number of individuals. One of the two drugs has since been withdrawn from the market, but the other, phentermine, is still considered to be proper and acceptable for aiding the dieter.

Your doctor will make the final decision as to whether this type of medication will be useful to you after a careful evaluation. I will only add that I prescribe such medications for many of my patients and I believe they can be quite helpful. Bear in mind that this type of medication is quite apart from the thyroid hormone I have discussed in this book. Appetite-suppressing medication may indeed be prescribed for those with hypothyroidism or those without.

Summing Up

- A reader with normal thyroid function should be able to lose weight effectively by following the diet presented in this book.
- A reader whose thyroid function is determined to be low by the MFI test results will need the assistance of a physician to correct the problem.
- The reader is instructed how best to approach the physician with the results of the testing.
- Anyone, whether hypothyroid or not, should diet under the supervision of his or her physician.

15

For Your Doctor's Eyes Only

Doctor,

You have probably been asked to read this chapter by one of your patients. It is quite possible that he or she has just completed the test in this book and there may be a question regarding the state of the patient's thyroid. This chapter is actually a summary of the entire book *Is Your Thyroid Making You Fat?* and should suffice to give you a good idea of my position on testing for hypothyroidism as well as the treatment. I would, of course, be honored if you would read the entire book, but I know how demanding a medical practice can be, and it is my hope that you will at least read this chapter.

I have limited my practice to the treatment of obesity for many years; in fact the millennium year will mark my fortieth year of dealing solely with overweight problems. My multiple offices have seen hundreds of thousands of patients during that time, and I don't need to tell you what a learning experience comes out of that type of repetition in a rather narrow field of interest.

The subject of the thyroid comes up with at least half of my patients, and it isn't I who introduces the subject. Many patients suspect they have an underactive thyroid, and they may actually state it in those terms. Quite frequently they allude obliquely to the suspicion that all isn't right with them by telling me they have something wrong with their bodies, that they cannot lose weight on the same diets that work for everyone else. They may even use the term *metabolism,* though frequently they use it incorrectly. A smaller number are much more knowledgeable. They know about hypothyroidism, and they know the various symptoms that may accompany it. The Internet has certainly become a tool of education in this area. What has frustrated them is that a doctor has tested them and told them there is nothing wrong with their thyroid gland.

This latter type of patient is often discontented with the diagnosis and even angry with the practitioner. They suspect that he distrusts the history of their eating habits they've given him. They don't like the implication that they are lying. This doesn't lend itself to a good doctor-patient relationship.

If we consider the two possibilities—one, that the patient is telling the truth and is eating a meager diet, and the other, that the patient is a liar and eats excessive amounts—it should be obvious that only one is consistent with a normal metabolism. My own experience, if not my own common sense, tells me that not all of these patients whose thyroid gland tests normal but who profess to eat reasonably can be lying. If some are telling the truth, it should be obvious that, at least in their case, there seems to be a deficiency of thyroid hormone. If there is any other reason for the phenomenon, I can't find it in the literature.

What then can we conclude from this? My conclusion is that lab testing doesn't demonstrate the deficiency of thyroid hormone in some patients. Does the lab ever help in the diagnosis of hypothyroidism? Obviously, yes. There are probably millions of people who take levothyroxine as a result of laboratory testing, and their symptoms are improved or even abated. If we conclude that laboratory testing sometimes demonstrates hypothyroidism and at other times misses it, how valuable is the lab in assisting with the diagnosis?

I'm reminded of a test that was popular a few years ago. It was a saliva test done on a pregnant woman to determine the sex of her unborn child. It was given in stores that sold maternity clothes or infants' clothes. The manufacturer of the test guaranteed accuracy by refunding the fee if it turned out that the results were in error. My guess is that they ended up keeping half of the fees.

I think there's an analogy there, but we're dealing with a more serious subject. If I can't rely on a test to have an accuracy of at least 90 percent, how can I rely on it at all? Even if I accept that hypothetical 90 percent figure and act accordingly, am I not potentially ignoring a serious medical problem in 1 out of 10 patients I've tested? The fact is that doctors rely so heavily on the lab results of the TSH and perhaps the T3 and T4, and occasionally a few other tests, that they don't seem to consider any other evidence. You might want to ask yourself this question: Under what circumstances would I start a patient on thyroid medication if the laboratory gave me no indication of a thyroid problem?

My own experience in performing these tests on patients was essentially a disaster. I believed the tests were accurate, and I was very reluctant to question what was so universally accepted. I shudder to think how many patients saw in my facial expression the belief that they were lying about their food consumption. What strengthened my cynicism were the occasions when I would test the same patient several days in a row and get such broadly varying results that I couldn't come to any conclusions. I won't even dwell on the few times I tested the lab by dividing the same blood specimen in half and sending it to the lab under two different names, only to receive the most disturbing results.

Obviously, my experience comes from a multitude of individual anecdotes about my patients. This isn't the usual way medical phenomena are reported. I don't have a university sponsor to add prestige to my findings. I am a practicing physician. I don't receive grants from pharmaceutical giants to fund my observations. Food companies don't subsidize my research, and the government agencies that fund research haven't paid me one cent. Yes, my findings are what the medical literature sometimes tolerates as "anecdotal evidence." I have a lot of that.

Is not all research anecdotal? Is it all not simply a collection of many, many anecdotes organized in a coherent fashion so that the researcher can draw conclusions from it? That's what I've done, not with the help of mainframe computers, shameful grants, or a staff of eager medical students. But my conclusions are every bit as valid, in my mind, mainly because of the volume of information I've acquired.

Haven't you within your own practice come to conclusions about the diagnosis and treatment of patients that are born of your own observations and experience and that are divergent from the mainstream of medical thought? That's exactly what I've done. I can't deny my observations or the conclusions I've drawn from them. I think I have a right to these conclusions. Forty years. Thousands of patients.

There is a monthly medical publication I receive called the *Cortlandt Forum.* Each issue devotes a substantial portion to short segments of anecdotal gems that come from practicing physicians around the country. I've found them to be a treasure of information. I'm not sure this kind of grass-roots research is worth much less than the ivory-tower variety.

My Test

We all know the multitude of signs and symptoms associated with hypothyroidism. I'm sure you see your share of patients who have the typical puffy dry skin, who seem to do everything at a snail's pace, who are always cold, whose hair is thin, and who perhaps exhibit other telltale signs. I imagine that you proceed to order a TSH and maybe some other tests. Perhaps the cholesterol is elevated, and perhaps by reflex you envision the patient gobbling down globs of saturated fat. When the TSH comes back and it's normal, what do you do? That dilemma frustrated me for years.

Because of my lack of confidence in the help I was getting from the lab, I had to look for other means. I knew full well that each hypothyroid patient didn't have every last one of the twenty-five or so signs associated with the ailment. Yet there is one common denominator, a factor that is inherent in the function of thyroid hormone. That single element is the inability of the patient to burn calories at the same rate as the euthyroid individual.

Over the years there have been a number of methods designed to measure the rate at which we use calories. I suspect that all suffer from the fact that the method itself introduces error into the calculation by actually changing the metabolic rate while the patient is undergoing testing. Years ago, I routinely did a basal metabolic rate test using a machine that measured inspired oxygen and expired carbon dioxide. That method fell out of favor a number of years ago because it was said to make the patient apprehensive and thus influence the outcome of the test.

The BMR test was replaced in many physicians' offices with Achilles reflex testing, a machine we would hook up to our EKG to use it as a recording device. We would tap the Achilles tendon on the kneeling patient and make a tracing, which would demonstrate the time lag in the recovery from the ankle jerk after the tap. We had a set of standards to compare the patient's response to some normal response. I actually liked the test, and it was generally right on when it came to substantiating the patient's signs and symptoms. Achilles reflex testing was eventually abandoned as the blood tests became more sophisticated and supposedly more accurate.

I've said that I believe the only common denominator of all hypothyroid patients is the substandard burning of calories. In a sense they have a more efficient engine than the norm; they seem to get more miles per gallon out of their calories. I expect you to now interject the question, "Why, then, aren't all hypothyroid patients overweight?"

The answer is inherent in what it is that makes us overweight. We become overweight when we ingest more calories than our system needs. The normal or underweight hypothyroid individual must be taking in a smaller number of calories than is normal. This is understandable. All of us aren't gluttons who will eat until the tank will hold no more. There are people who aren't that much into food. They can either take it or leave it, and usually they leave it. Thus, on an intake of calories that would result in most people losing weight, they do not lose. They simply maintain their weight.

As soon as I accepted the fact that this slow metabolism was the universal factor, it didn't seem very difficult to measure it. We have a wealth of useful data. During the first half of the twentieth century, there was much research in developing methods for determining our caloric needs. Various formulas were devised, the most well-known of which is the Harris-Benedict formula. It has been massaged, critiqued, and supposedly improved over the years, and it is still used to calculate caloric needs, particularly of patients who must be fed involuntarily, such as comatose patients or the elderly. Various factors enter into the calculation: age, sex, frame size, etc. These calculations lead to a value for the baseline metabolism of the individual. By applying factors that correct for various activity levels, we can come up with an intelligent guess as to how many calories a "normal" individual needs in order to maintain his or her weight, in other words, the corrected caloric maintenance level, which for convenience I've dubbed the CCML.

The test I've devised and which I use in my practice involves monitoring the patient's calorie intake over a fixed period of time and also noting the weight change during that same period. We know that each pound of weight lost represents a caloric deficit of 3,500 calories. Since we know the total caloric deficit for the period, we divide this number by the number of days represented and we arrive at the average daily caloric deficit. We know (1) how many calories the reader (or the patient) consumed during the test period, and (2) what the weight loss was during that period. By adding the two, we have the number of calories that would have maintained the weight of the individual during the diet period. By dividing that number by the number of days the person dieted, we arrive at the daily corrected caloric maintenance level (CCML) for that individual.

By dividing the actual maintenance level by the standard (expected) maintenance level, then multiplying by 100, we come up with a percentage of normal. I've boldly named this percentage the Metabolic Function Index (MFI). (I couldn't bring myself to name it the Siegal index.)

As an example, if an individual should require 2,000 calories per day to maintain her weight and the testing she had done shows that she would maintain her weight eating 1,400 calories per day, her MFI is 70 percent. My experience tells me that she is hypothyroid. I arbitrarily regard 90 percent as the cutoff point, mainly because there is certainly room for error in the calculations. Below that number is some degree of hypothyroidism.

The method I use is unique, but not bizarre. It gets right to the heart of the matter and it doesn't rely upon a distant laboratory for its accuracy. True, my readers need to have done everything correctly and I've emphasized this in these pages, but since they have a direct interest in the outcome, I suspect the average reader will expend great effort to see that the results are valid. I actually think readers of this book will produce a more valid result than will my own patients who believe I'm sitting in judgment of their deeds. The reader has to answer only to herself or himself.

If you question the validity of such an exercise as I've described, ask yourself, What could cause this substandard loss of fat other than insufficient thyroid hormone? Assuming that there isn't a lot of fluid retention on the day the test ended or that there isn't extreme dehydration, I believe the conclusions are valid. Readers are cautioned to be alert for the possibility of fluid retention.

The true weakness of the test is that it relies on the honesty of the patient. I wouldn't be surprised if patients sometimes deceive me about their straying from the diet because of embarrassment. As I've said, I think they are less likely to lie to themselves when they are taking the test in this book. I've tried to impress upon my readers the virtues of honesty.

There are two other "tests" the reader is asked to take. One involves simply taking one's temperature on arising. It is based on the common knowledge that those with hypothyroidism generally run a lower body temperature than those with normal thyroid function. If you exclude times when the reader is ovulating or when she has an infection, you can form an impression of whether the body temperature points to a low metabolic rate. A doctor by the name of Broda Barnes wrote a book in 1976 in which he espoused the belief that this was *the* test for hypothyroidism. The book is still in print after all these years. This must attest to the fact that there are people who still want to know what he had to say. He, like me, wasn't enamored with the usual laboratory testing. I've asked my readers to take serial temperature readings as sort of a corroboration of what the MFI test reveals.

A second corroborating test is based simply on the reader asking questions of himself or herself. The idea is to see if the reader has the signs and symptoms that are prevalent in hypothyroidism. The questions are adapted from a 1969 study in which a group of Scottish researchers attempted to develop a practical method of diagnosing hypothyroidism that wasn't invasive. What made their test unique was the clever weighting method they assigned to each symptom and that a positive or negative answer weren't necessarily weighted equally.* I can tell you that when I see a new patient with a hoarse, raspy voice who obviously moves very slowly and who tells me she never sweats, I suspect hypothyroidism, and I will be right much more often than wrong.

Thyroid Medication

Today's standard treatment of hypothyroidism is almost universally the prescribing of levothyroxine. This, as you know, is one of the thyroid hormones and is the one that is secreted in the greatest quantity. It is often abbreviated as T4, and for brevity I shall use that designation. I would guess that at least 90 percent

---

*Billewicz, W. Z., et al., "Statistical Methods Applied to the Diagnosis of Hypothyroidism," *Quarterly Journal of Medicine,* New Series XXXVIII, No. 150, April 1969, pp. 255–266.

of the thyroid hormone prescribed in this country is T4, although T3 (triiodothyronine) is sometimes prescribed. Even less frequent is the prescription of desiccated thyroid.

Desiccated thyroid has various synonyms, among them Thyroid U.S.P., which is probably the most proper. Frequently it is called Armour Thyroid and sometimes simply Armour because of its long-term association with the Armour meat company that was the source of the animal thyroid glands used to make the product. Repeatedly in this book, I've referred to it as "natural thyroid," which distinguishes it from synthetic T4.

If you're a lot younger than I, you may only vaguely know of the existence of Thyroid U.S.P., since its use fell off dramatically with the introduction of synthetic T4 in the 1950s. It is still a United States Pharmacopeia drug, and virtually all pharmacies stock it.

You may have guessed that I've devoted these previous paragraphs to this explanation for more than a history lesson. The fact is that I prefer the use of Thyroid U.S.P. to synthetic T4. The reason for this is as simple as it gets: I find that it works better.

More history may help to explain my position: The first use of thyroid hormone in humans dates back to 1891, when a doctor by the name of Murray crudely extracted some soup from sheep thyroid glands and injected it into a myxedematous patient with a remarkable outcome. He reported his findings with the usual degree of British understatement in the *British Medical Journal.* Within a very short time others realized they could achieve the same effect by giving sheep thyroid orally. For the next fifty years or so, hypothyroidism was treated with essentially that method.

For the first fifty years of the 1900s, desiccated thyroid was virtually the only choice. It was prescribed widely and essentially controlled hypothyroidism admirably. Its use wasn't without criticism. From time to time there were complaints from physicians as well as patients that subsequent prescriptions of it didn't seem to have the same therapeutic effect as the previous one. It was suggested that the potency was quite variable and that the physician could not rely upon the strength printed on the label. One explanation is that the product lost potency on the pharmacy shelves and there was little regulation of matters dealing with shelf life. Its reputation wasn't helped by an incident involving unscrupulous suppliers importing a large quantity of a totally bogus substance.

When synthetic T4 became available in the fifties, it was believed to be much more stable on the shelf and therefore more reliable as to dosage. The reasoning was that even though our own thyroid glands produce both T4 and T3, the former is converted within us to T3 anyway, so why bother giving the mixture. I, like many other physicians, began switching my patients from Thyroid U.S.P. to synthetic T4. I must point out that I had never had the experience of the erratic potency that had been reported but, always willing to keep up with the times, I began changing my patients over to T4.

Almost immediately I began to hear complaints. Patients would report a lethargy that was something new. Weight loss in a number of patients was noticeably decreased. In short, many symptoms of hypothyroidism seemed to be increasing. Patients themselves expressed dissatisfaction by making comments like "Why did you change my medicine?" or, more directly, "This new stuff you gave me is no good."

I never did switch the whole practice over to T4, but I was also not that quick in going back to Thyroid U.S.P. in those who had been switched. I was skeptical as to my own observations and as to what was being reported to me by patients. Who was I to doubt the most recent medical dicta?

Another frequently repeated scenario starts with a patient who comes to me having previously been diagnosed as hypothyroid and who is already taking synthetic T4 prescribed by another doctor. At the point when I began to doubt the efficacy of T4, I would often switch the patient from T4 to Thyroid U.S.P. The change was often dramatic. Almost without exception I could see an improvement. There were those patients who reported that previously their doctors had reduced the amount of synthetic T4 they had been taking because of annoying side effects, such as increased blood pressure, fast pulse rate, or even tremors. I've rarely seen the same effect from comparable doses of Thyroid U.S.P.

Eventually I abandoned T4, and for years I've been prescribing Thyroid U.S.P. exclusively and I'm quite satisfied with the results. To repeat the simple answer to the question of why I prescribe Thyroid U.S.P.: *Because it works better.*

The bloom began to disappear from the rose when the potency of the widely dispensed synthetic T4 was brought into question. In 1997 the government dictated that although levothyroxine had been marketed for years, because of inconsistent stability and potency manufacturers would be required to submit new drug applications (NDAs) for the product. The following is actual wording from the *Federal Register:*

> No currently marketed orally administered levothyroxine sodium product has been shown to demonstrate consistent potency and stability and, thus, no currently marketed orally administered levothyroxine sodium product is generally recognized as safe and effective.

The very complaints that for years had plagued the prescribing of Thyroid U.S.P. now seemed at least as applicable to synthetic thyroid.

I have essentially told my readers the story I've just told you. They may be asking you to prescribe Thyroid U.S.P. I hope the previous explanation will be helpful to you as you make this decision.

A paper published in *The New England Journal of Medicine* in February 1999 served to strengthen my belief. This book was well into preparation at that time, and I was pleased to be able to support my beliefs by alluding to that study. Researchers found that substituting T3 for some of the T4 hypothyroid patients were receiving produced a better result than did T4 alone. Thyroid U.S.P. contains both T3 and T4.

Whether you choose to try Thyroid U.S.P. on some patients is a choice you may decide to make. I would expect that if you do, your experience will be much like mine.

In my conversations with other doctors regarding patients under our joint care, I've frequently been asked why I use such an obscure drug. (They believe it to be obscure.) Can you imagine how many times I've had to go through the explanation I've just given you?

You're certainly aware of the paradox that exists between the degree of ignorance of some patients and the remarkable degree of knowledge of others. In this electronic age, we can't underestimate the astuteness of our patients. Thyroid patients' comments are very conspicuous on an excellent Web site devoted to the entire subject of thyroid disorders (thyroid.about.com). Of interest is a letter posted by a patient. It is to her doctor, and it is poignantly critical of his refusal to prescribe Thyroid U.S.P. for her.

I will get down to how I initiate treatment on a patient whose MFI tells me she doesn't burn calories at the normal rate. I give the patient a trial of Thyroid U.S.P. A frequent starting dose is ½ grain daily. In many instances that isn't sufficient, and I see the patient frequently and observe her as well as listen to her subjective reports. If I am 99 percent certain of hypothyroidism, I may start with 1 grain. My routine is to increase the dosage by ½ grain no more often than once a month when the signs and symptoms seem to warrant it. In every case, I monitor the amount by how the patient looks and feels and by what she reports to me. Remember, the patient is in my office primarily to lose weight, and it was the observation of the rate of weight loss that resulted in the assessment of hypothyroidism. Thus, weight loss is one of the more important determinants of my thyroid dosage. I would always prefer to err on the side of conservatism, and so a reasonable but not spectacular rate of weight loss is what I seek. The general overall state of well-being of the patient is even a greater influence in the judgment I make.

For the majority of the patients I see who have hypothyroidism, 1 to 1½ grains of Thyroid U.S.P. seems to be the proper dose. In some instances, I go higher. Except in the most rare of cases, perhaps 1 or 2 patients in my entire practice, I haven't had to exceed 3 grains, although in the literature much higher doses have been reported to have been needed.

Thyroid for the Euthyroid Patient

It has been some years since thyroid medication has been advocated as a weight-loss tool. In the past it was used extensively without regard to the thyroid status of the individual receiving it. Searching the literature, I haven't found conclusive evidence that using thyroid for weight loss was ever harmful, although there is certainly enough opinion that it should not be done.

I have had no personal experience with prescribing thyroid to the euthyroid patient. I prescribe it after I determine that the patient needs it. However, if the standard for determining who is hypothyroid are the chemical laboratory tests, then indeed I could be accused of giving thyroid to a euthyroid patient. Of course, whether I'm guilty in the eyes of those doing the accusing might depend upon what day they did their tests. The point is that I've never seen anyone suffer harm from thyroid medication unless it was an obvious allergy, such as an urticaria. I explain this by reasoning that the thyroid was needed by those for whom I prescribed it.

As long as the standard remains the results of lab testing, I cannot evaluate the literature with any sense of accomplishing anything. The scientific literature in general assigns the diagnosis of hypothyroidism to those with an elevated TSH. If the baseline is what I consider to be an erroneous assumption, how can I draw valid conclusions? Totally disregarded are the signs and symptoms the patient presents as well as the obvious inappropriate response to what should be a deficiency of calories in the diet.

The question of whether thyroid medication, irrespective of thyroid disease, is an appropriate treatment for obesity is one that should be researched. I haven't prescribed thyroid in that instance, and I'm not about to embark on such a research project.

Given the general apathy toward the whole subject, I also have my doubts as to whether anyone else will. [There is more about this concept in Appendix A.]

Emphasis on Protein

In recent years there has been a dramatic shift in what is considered the best type of diet to follow. We now have the Food Pyramid, which displays a suggested diet of a considerable amount of carbohydrate, little fat, and a small amount of protein. This expresses the general dietary recommendations of what "experts" have been advocating for years. This has been applied not just to general diet, but also to reducing diets. Prior to that and extending back to the middle of the nineteenth century, a diet high in protein and relatively low in carbohydrate was considered to be the ideal reducing diet. There were plenty of published studies to substantiate that a high-protein diet produced the best weight-loss result.

It is my observation that the obesity problem has become more widespread and more severe with the current emphasis upon carbohydrate. Of course I'm not alone. Very recently there have been a host of books and magazine articles singing the praises of the high-protein diet. Some advocate very high fat at the same time, and this has been severely criticized. Fat in the diet adds much to the satisfying quality of food and it does slow the gastric emptying time. Whether those factors justify the added nine calories per gram or the possible dangers aren't matters that I will address here. But, at the moment, protein seems to be in.

I have always felt that the high-protein diet was the best for my patients. Like many other aspects of my practice, what I do with my patients is based upon what seems to serve them best. I've had a lot of years to observe the effects of various techniques, and I've had a lot of patients on whom to make these observations. The bottom line is that my patients get the best results when they eat a high-protein diet.

We could debate whether this is due to the specific dynamic action of protein. This concept is well established and has never been disproved, but it is for the most part ignored. Quite simply, protein digestion and assimilation requires a greater expenditure of calories by the body than does carbohydrate or fat. [There is more about this in Chapter 9.]

At any rate, my reason for advocating protein is much like the reason I like the metabolic test I use and the medication I prefer: *They simply work better.*

The Diet

The diet I've advocated in this book is designed to work. I've avoided the gimmicks and nonsense that accompany so many of the magic diets out there. What I advise is what I've found the majority of patients can follow. The diet has no magic. It is designed to meet the needs of the majority of my readers.

I like the 1,000-calorie level. In my own practice, more frequently I advocate 800. I'm comfortable with it and I try to get patients to make weekly visits in order to monitor it. Some cannot tolerate that few calories and so I must go up to 1,000 or more, and the weight loss is slightly slower. By the same token, I've found no advantage in going too much lower than 800 calories. Below that, the metabolic rate probably falls and weight loss slows, so there really is no advantage. Furthermore, it confuses the hypothyroidism situation and makes adjusting the thyroid dose more of a task. Of course, this is your patient and you must decide on the diet. If you aren't comfortable with 1,000 calories or the emphasis on protein, certainly other combinations will work as long as the calories are restricted. A few calories more will still result in weight loss, even if at a slower rate. The important thing is to encourage the patient to reach the goal that has been set. If the patients don't get to the target weight, rarely do they maintain the weight they've achieved. Invariably, they gain it back. I go to lengths to emphasize to my patients that they must get to the goal weight that has been set for them.

I make free use of packaged foods, frozen, canned, or otherwise. I tend to ask my patients to stick with foods for which they can easily determine the calorie count. There are enough of these to keep them interested. Packaged foods have the calorie counts clearly stated, and for many of the bulk foods I've provided the necessary caloric information. One of the calorie books I've recommended can come in handy.

I'm quite flexible about how the reader is permitted to exercise options. Three meals a day isn't an absolute requirement. The lifestyle of many allows only two, and the individual is often quite comfortable with that. Likewise, the distribution of calories between the meals doesn't seem all that important. I've seen no proof that it makes a bit of difference. So whether it is a bigger breakfast or a bigger dinner isn't material. The important item is the calorie count. If you stress the importance of that, neither you nor they can go wrong.

Without a doubt, the average patient will have fewer or less productive bowel movements when eating 1,000 calories a day, down from the customary 3,000. This is the basis for a frequent complaint. It is generally reported as constipation, but I reserve that term for times when the patient is truly physically uncomfortable. Some people are perhaps overly concerned about having a daily bowel movement, and my insistence on a high-fiber cereal for breakfast probably contributes to their peace of mind.

The Patient May Need Your Cooperation

The patient's basic motivation is the major factor in whether the whole exercise turns out to be a success or a fiasco. A close second on the list of what helps is the encouragement given by the caregiver, in this case, you. I believe you must continually support, encourage, warn, and, in some cases, criticize, but in every case you need to convey the impression that you expect the patient to achieve a normal weight. You must nurse them through the times when they've followed the instructions scrupulously and have for a week or so shown no weight loss. As far as the scale is concerned, even in the most rigid adherents, weight does not come off a little each day. It comes off in spurts, sometimes intermingled with weight gain. You, as well as the patient, should have faith in the science. Quite simply, an adult human cannot continually eat 1,000 calories a day over the long haul and not lose weight.

Contact me. I would love to hear from you. Perhaps you have questions. I will answer them to the best of my ability. The best means to contact me is through my Web site. The address is: www.drsiegal.com.

16

Debating My Position

I don't resent criticism, even when, for the sake of emphasis, it parts for the time with reality.
—*Winston Churchill*

The methods of diagnosis and treatment I've described in these pages are assuredly different from what you've been exposed to in the past. Perhaps you've been told you have normal thyroid function based on laboratory work that was done, and perhaps I've raised some questions in your mind that maybe it's just not so. Perhaps you already know you have hypothyroidism and are being treated with synthetic thyroid hormone, but I've cast some doubt on whether you're getting the optimal treatment. Perhaps you're having difficulty losing weight and are wondering whether the methods I've described in this book will really work for you.

If these concepts seem contrary to what you've been told in the past, you must understand that they will seem even more divergent to the majority of doctors who read this book or hear about it. Doctors aren't shy when it comes to voicing opinions. I know that by the time you read this, you will have heard contrary opinions. I don't know how severe the criticism will be, but I do know it will be there. I also expect some degree of approval from a number of physicians who have had the same type of experiences with their patients that I've had with mine. I even hope to enlist some converts who will at least consider seriously what I've reported here and implement some of these ideas into their medical practices.

True debates over new ideas of this type often make their way into the media. Yet it would be rare for the public ever to have the benefit of a full-scale debate that covers both sides of an issue. What you will generally get is a one-sided declaration from some authority. If the authority happens to be me, it will obviously be one-sided because, as fair as I wish to be with my critics, I believe what I believe, and as I've said before, my experience is what has shaped my opinions. If the authority is another doctor, he also has a right to his opinions. That's what a debate is for. Both sides can be expressed freely and the audience can decide. But the likelihood of a full-scale debate is slim.

Since I anticipate some one-sided criticism, perhaps from your own doctor, and perhaps from articles in newspapers or magazines or perhaps on TV or radio, I've decided to reproduce such a debate here. I will fairly represent the criticism of what I have to say, and I will respond to it. I believe I know most of the arguments that will be used, and I believe I can express them fairly.

Here is a mythical confrontation between the noted thyroid authority, whom I shall name Dr. I. M. Conformist, and Dr. Siegal.

DR. CONFORMIST: Thank you for meeting with me, Dr. Siegal. I've been reading from your book. I found it interesting, but there is much I would like to discuss with you.

DR. SIEGAL: I welcome your interest.

DR. CONFORMIST: As you certainly are aware, some of the concepts you've expressed seem to be directly in conflict with what is generally accepted as standard when it comes to the treatment of hypothyroidism. Are you not troubled by that?

DR. SIEGAL: I'm not troubled by it, but I would prefer not to find it necessary to disagree with so much current thought in this area. However, that is the reason for this book. I can't ignore what my patients have taught me. The reason for this book is that I do disagree. I believe that what I've presented here can be very useful to my readers. My secret hope is that it will foster more research in this area.

DR. CONFORMIST: I have no problem with your recognition of the signs and symptoms of hypothyroidism, although you do seem to think it is more prevalent than what is generally believed. But you do seem to be quite critical of the standard methods of diagnosis, methods that are universally accepted.

DR. SIEGAL: Yes, they are widely accepted, but I don't accept them. I believe there are a number of other doctors who don't. It's been over twenty-five years since Dr. Barnes wrote his book on the subject, and I happen to agree with much of what he had to say. Do you know that his book is still in print? That's unusual for a popular medical book. It must have made an impression on readers who could relate to what he had to say. Most books of that type are usually gone from the bookstores in a few months.

DR. CONFORMIST: I've heard of Dr. Barnes's book, but I must confess I haven't read it.

DR. SIEGAL: Dr. Barnes criticized the practice of diagnosing thyroid problems through the use of the laboratory. He felt that the diagnosis of hypothyroidism was often missed by physicians who had too much confidence in the laboratory. That has also been my experience.

DR. CONFORMIST: Why are you so negative on thyroid tests such as the TSH?

DR. SIEGAL: It seems that most doctors accept lab results even when they seem to be in conflict with their own observations. We all know that labs can make mistakes, and no one berates them for it. What I'm speaking of is quite different. I believe that tests such as the TSH, even when done flawlessly, miss the diagnosis of hypothyroidism quite frequently. What is my evidence for this? Many patients I've seen and whom I believed to have hypothyroidism had normal laboratory values. As soon as they started taking thyroid hormone, their symptoms abated. They showed no ill effects on later follow-up. Is this not persuasive evidence of my position? Much of the research that's done starts with the premise that the lab tests are infallible. If, for example, you wished to test a medication only on hypothyroid patients but you excluded some from the study because it was determined from the lab that they weren't candidates, in my opinion, you would have a flawed experiment.

DR. CONFORMIST: The TSH test is the first step in investigating thyroid function, whether overactive or underactive. Yet you say you have no confidence in it.

DR. SIEGAL: I've done thousands of thyroid tests on my patients over the years, TSH and others. As I look back, I realize they were virtually of no help in aiding in the diagnosis of hypothyroidism.

DR. CONFORMIST: The medical community disagrees: I use the test regularly with my patients and I uncover many cases of hypothyroidism.

DR. SIEGAL: I'm certain you do. My concern isn't with those that are discovered, it is with those that go undiscovered. Do you think some slip by?

DR. CONFORMIST: I'm sure that has happened on a few occasions and those were probably borderline cases, so-called subclinical hypothyroidism.

DR. SIEGAL: How do you know you haven't missed many more cases?

DR. CONFORMIST: Because I have tested my patients and the tests have shown me who has the ailment and who doesn't.

DR. SIEGAL: But that is exactly my point. You rely on the test results exclusively. What if the tests are flawed?

DR. CONFORMIST: The medical community didn't accept these tests without a lot of research to back them up. We have to trust the scientists.

DR. SIEGAL: I do trust them, but I can't ignore what I've seen with my own eyes. Do you ever see patients who have multiple symptoms of hypothyroidism but the TSH comes back normal or even low?

DR. CONFORMIST: Yes, that happens sometimes.

DR. SIEGAL: How do you account for it?

DR. CONFORMIST: The patient has normal thyroid function and therefore I must look elsewhere for the cause of the patient's symptoms.

DR. SIEGAL: With this type of patient, are you usually successful in finding the cause of their symptoms?

DR. CONFORMIST: Sometimes yes and sometimes no. As you know, we doctors aren't always successful in arriving at a diagnosis. Some ailments simply defy discovery.

DR. SIEGAL: Would you consider treating a patient for hypothyroidism if she had all the symptoms but the laboratory said she didn't have the ailment?

DR. CONFORMIST: I won't say I would never do it, but it would be a rare occasion.

DR. SIEGAL: If, on one of those rare occasions, you prescribed thyroid hormone and there was a dramatic improvement in the patient's condition, would you continue the treatment?

DR. CONFORMIST: Yes, I suppose so.

DR. SIEGAL: This is essentially what I'm doing, except it seems to happen with greater frequency. It appears that the only difference you and I have so far is when it comes to confidence in certain specific lab results.

DR. CONFORMIST: So you are saying that you've had a number of patients who test normal but actually have hypothyroidism?

DR. SIEGAL: Yes, literally thousands over the last forty years. I haven't kept track of the numbers.

DR. CONFORMIST: But how do you know you haven't been prescribing thyroid hormone to patients who have normal thyroid function?

DR. SIEGAL: The patient tells me. If there is a clear-cut reversal of the symptoms, I can only conclude that I was correct. The patient knows. I think we have to listen to our patients. If my patient changes from an apathetic recluse to a socially competent individual and at the same time her periods straighten out, her depression vanishes, and she is able to lose weight for the first time in her life, then I have to assume that I was correct. And if her hopeless infertility for which she's spent thousands of dollars on diagnosis and treatment ends in a pregnancy two months after starting on thyroid hormone, then I'm even more certain that I was right.

DR. CONFORMIST: You ask the readers to take this test of yours. A doctor would have to have a lot of confidence in your method to ignore the laboratory in favor of your test.

DR. SIEGAL: I have confidence in the method because over the years it has served me better than the lab has in this area. You understand this isn't a blanket condemnation of laboratory tests. My complaint specifically targets thyroid tests. As to whether a doctor will try my test and accept the results, I hope I've made a good case for trying it. If after hearing the patient's history he is convinced she has a weight problem in spite of her moderate eating habits, I hope he will entertain the possibility of hypothyroidism. I expect the doctor to listen to everything the patient says and assume that he is hearing the truth unless there is some special reason to doubt what the patient has said.

The history tells me a lot. Are you aware of the questionnaire that is part of the testing? It is quite valuable. It was adapted from a well-known study aimed at finding an alternate and perhaps more cost-effective means of diagnosing hypothyroidism.

What about the patient's body temperature? Don't you agree that a low body temperature, though not definitive, is certainly consistent with hypothyroidism? And what about a high blood cholesterol? I've seen one case after another of patients whose cholesterol was brought under control where there was nothing to account for the improvement except for the thyroid hormone they had been prescribed.

There are other doctors who believe just as I do, but they are simply not vocal. More importantly, there are intelligent and perplexed patients who feel the same way. Do you know that there is a Web site where patients air their complaints against doctors who ignore their hypothyroidism? They regularly post messages asking others to find them a doctor who will look beyond lab results.

DR. CONFORMIST: Let's move on. I noticed that you prescribe desiccated thyroid for your hypothyroid patients. I run into desiccated thyroid every now and then, and when a new patient has been taking it, I usually switch her over to levothyroxine (synthetic thyroid). I don't know anyone who prescribes desiccated thyroid anymore.

DR. SIEGAL: I do. And I do it for one simple reason: It works better. That's not to say that synthetic thyroid doesn't work, but natural thyroid works better. By the way, I like to call it "natural thyroid" in order to avoid confusion with the synthesized varieties.

DR. CONFORMIST: Has it not been established that the strength of what you call natural thyroid is inconsistent and that the potency can vary considerably?

DR. SIEGAL: I've researched the subject completely. I find no documentation that natural thyroid is unreliable, even though I've heard that rumor. I do know that it was actually the potency of synthetic thyroid that was questioned by the FDA and serious sanctions were imposed on the manufacturers. Keep in mind that after all these years, natural thyroid is still a U.S.P. drug, as is levothyroxine sodium. In a recent book by Dr. Arem, a recognized thyroid expert, he recounts how some of his patients, when he switches them from natural to synthetic, complain. They tell him it doesn't work as well. He, however, seems unconvinced. Unlike Dr. Arem, I am convinced. Perhaps I've heard it more often than he has. I've dealt with the problem so frequently over the years that there is no question about it in my mind. Natural thyroid works better than the synthetic levothyroxine. Have you prescribed much desiccated thyroid?

DR. CONFORMIST: No. As long as I have been in practice, the literature has specified levothyroxine as the drug of choice.

DR. SIEGAL: That is certainly the case. You're speaking of synthetic thyroid. I wonder how many doctors would change their minds if they were to prescribe natural thyroid for some of their patients and see the results I've seen. On that same Web site I mentioned earlier, the one where thyroid patients commiserate with one another, one of the most frequent complaints is that some doctor took them off the natural thyroid that worked for them and they cannot find another doctor who will prescribe it. They plead for the name of a doctor who will help them.

I believe that the reason for the popularity of synthetic thyroid has more to do with marketing than any other factor. We doctors are bombarded with advertising, and it must certainly shape our prescribing tendencies, otherwise why would the drug companies spend so much money trying to get us to prescribe their products?

DR. CONFORMIST: I have the impression that you use thyroid hormone as a weight-loss medication.

DR. SIEGAL: Absolutely not. I don't prescribe thyroid hormone unless I'm convinced the patient has hypothyroidism. In those cases, it isn't for weight loss, but to correct the thyroid problem. But in the course of doing that, it may indeed help the weight loss because now the metabolism is brought up closer to normal. We may someday learn that it can be used for weight loss in the patient who isn't hypothyroid, but so far I haven't done it.

DR. CONFORMIST: As to your MFI test, I haven't heard of any testing that used a patient's caloric maintenance level as a basis for the diagnosis of hypothyroidism.

DR. SIEGAL: To my knowledge, it hasn't been done before. Isn't it logical that the number of calories that maintain a patient's weight is intimately connected with how the thyroid functions? Do you have some reason to believe it isn't accurate? Suppose a patient of yours is on a 1,000-calorie diet and in a month loses only 2 pounds. That translates into that patient maintaining her weight on 1,250 calories a day. What other explanation could there be for this other than hypothyroidism?

DR. CONFORMIST: I don't know. There could be some other hormonal imbalance. Maybe she is retaining a lot of fluid. Maybe she's stretched the truth a bit.

DR. SIEGAL: I look for other explanations, such as the water retention you mentioned. It's not difficult to detect. The point is, Doctor, that is how I make the diagnosis of hypothyroidism. If the patient doesn't burn calories at the same rate as someone with normal thyroid function, I call that hypothyroidism. It's really quite simple. Besides, the important thing isn't what you call their signs and symptoms, but rather what you can do to alleviate them. When a patient presents me with such an underactive metabolism, it is almost a certainty that she has several other hypothyroid symptoms. If administering thyroid hormone makes her feel better and she starts losing weight, I'm satisfied with the name I've given her condition. In the end, the name isn't what is important, it is the welfare of the patient. There is no question that some patients will fudge about their eating habits, and I've become rather skilled at sensing when my patient isn't all that truthful. We have to be careful that we don't categorize patients as liars as a catchall for our frustrations. If we can't explain the reason for what the patient reports, it isn't always because we're being deceived.

DR. CONFORMIST: The diet you recommend for weight loss is slanted very much in the protein direction. It doesn't conform to the USDA's Food Pyramid.

DR. SIEGAL: It is my impression that the pyramid was intended as a guide to "proper eating" habits. I'm not sure that it is even proper for maintaining weight, although that is an entirely different subject. There is nothing proper about a diet for losing weight. To lose weight you must follow a deficient diet, one that is deficient in calories. I've chosen the high-protein diet for the same reason I've done all these other things, because it works. I've watched twenty years or more of this emphasis on carbohydrate in the diet and I've seen the obesity problem seriously worsen during that time. High protein, moderate carbohydrates, and very little fat results in weight loss with minimal hunger in a motivated patient.

DR. CONFORMIST: Doctor, your ideas are different. Is it good to shake patients' confidence in their physicians? This cannot be to their benefit.

DR. SIEGAL: I've agonized on this point. What would you do? You seem to be in disagreement with my ideas. Should you restrain yourself from criticizing me? These aren't my "ideas." These are the conclusions from my observations. I didn't simply read some scientific papers and put all the information in them together into a book. Everything I've reported is based upon my experience with thousands of patients. Should I not share this information?

I didn't really know how to end this interview. My position is clear, and it is unlikely that Dr. Conformist will withdraw from his. In the real world, the interview will probably end when the moderator says that it is time to take a commercial break.

If it seems unusual that I have taken the time to criticize my own work, so be it. I've done so because I believe there is the possibility that you will hear bits and pieces of the type of criticism I've described above. It is likely that any criticism will be one-sided, so in the interest of fairness or, more importantly, in your best interests, I've organized the criticism and have presented both sides.

My Web site is there for you, your doctor, and anyone else to use to communicate with me. You'll find me at www. drsiegal.com.

17

Maintaining Weight, Hypothyroid or Not

Sometime during the course of treatment of a patient, the subject of weight maintenance will come up. When a patient first begins the program, it seems perhaps too optimistic even to entertain that thought, but when it appears that the goal is in sight, how she will maintain a normal weight in the future becomes a real concern.

The vast majority of people who lose weight gain it back. This occurs in spite of the best intentions of the weight loser, let alone the lofty motives of those who facilitated that weight loss. It applies to my patients as well as to those who got their direction from some magazine article. Whether you join an organization that uses group enthusiasm to motivate you or you buy questionable packaged meals from one of those widely advertised "clinics," or even if you succeeded through the devoted efforts of your doctor, the fact is that the odds favor your gaining back what you've lost.

Strangely enough, my patients seem convinced that they will not regain the weight. "I will never again allow this to happen" seems to be the frequent slogan. The patient who proclaims this really believes that. But it does happen, and, what's more, she allows it to happen.

There is a certain sameness to all weight-maintenance efforts. One clinic presents a particular set of eating rules that will keep you thin for a lifetime. A book says to make sure you eat this much of this and that every day, but keep this and that below a certain amount. Your doctor may speak in terms of units of food or exchange groups. It all amounts to the same thing. Everyone says that the way to maintain your weight is to follow some sensible eating regime for the rest of your life. Who could fault such sage advice? Of course it will work. You eat what you're supposed to and you will never gain back your weight. That's obvious.

But virtually everyone does gain back the weight. Why? Because they don't follow that very fine advice. That is the rule. Anyone who does spend the rest of his days eating exactly what he's been told to is the rare exception.

My question to all concerned is, What good is it to pass out advice you know no one will follow? One answer is that it gets the advice-giver off the hook. If I tell my patient that for the rest of her life she must eat this and that and she disobeys me, I'm home free. But what about my conscience? What if, in my heart, I knew she would not follow that advice, in spite of the fact that she thought she would? What then? Can I still claim innocence?

This is the crux of the problem. There is a lot of good advice out there that no one follows. What's more, anyone who has dealt with overweight patients over the years knows that what I'm reporting is right on. Any doctor who has seen a few thousand overweight patients knows that once the weight is lost, it is easily regained in spite of the good intentions of the patient.

This knowledge is enough to make one throw up one's hands and look for a more satisfying job, like selling refrigerators in Antarctica. But there is one ray of hope.

Not all of my patients gain back the weight they have lost. There is a relatively small number who do maintain the weight, and possibly way into the foreseeable future. Two observations characterize this group.

Everyone who maintains weight long term seems to have first reached the goal weight that was set for them. I will tell you quickly that I don't really know the reason for this. But it does seem to be a fact, at least in my own practice. A patient may have lost one hundred pounds or so, yet still have another twenty or thirty to go. She may be so overjoyed at the change that she no longer perceives any kind of problem. I may emphasize to her that she is now at the stage when many patients first come to me. She now has twenty-five pounds to lose, and it is very common for a new patient to come in who has twenty-five pounds to lose. This doesn't seem to make an impression on certain people. The crisis of that first hundred pounds is over and she simply can't motivate herself further.

This is the patient who is certain to gain back the weight.

Whether the prerequisite of reaching the goal weight in order to increase the likelihood of permanent success is a physical or a psychological phenomenon is beyond my ability to investigate. I've repeatedly told you that I'm a practical kind of doctor; if it works, do it. If you don't know why it works, and it causes no harm, do it anyway. While the dedicated scientists are delving into the answers, I can help a lot of people.

My first admonition to a new patient is that she must achieve the goal weight that is determined for her. I even go so far as to say that she should not even start the program if the intention isn't to reach the goal. It will be a total waste of time and perhaps even be counterproductive.

This poses a problem with some of my patients, and it is generally the female patient. There are many women who don't want to be as thin as I want them to be. This group is usually in the fourth decade of life or beyond. Some honestly tell me that the concern is that they will look older. They know that as the fat layer disappears, the skin will become looser. The skin is being stretched and wrinkles are consequently minimal. They know that after losing weight they may begin to show their true age, and this isn't acceptable to them. I have a hard time convincing them otherwise. This matter of vanity seems to be far more powerful than the desire for health.

I've pointed out that at least in the case of females, one rather large study shows a straight-line relationship between what you weigh and how long you live. For those overly concerned about that loose skin, there seems to be little concern about how long they live. They just want to look their best. Of course, there are vast differences in the elastic qualities of skin in different individuals. In some, I've seen no hint that an enormous amount of weight has been lost, yet in others, it is quite obvious.

At any rate, my advice has to be predicated on my patient's health and not on how she stacks up to the ladies on the magazine covers. I insist that my patients reach the goal I set for them.

Though I'm sure that a proper weight is a requirement of weight maintenance, it isn't the only requirement. Getting to your goal weight isn't absolute insurance that you will stay there. A second factor is always present in my patients who maintain weight, and that is exercise. I never see anyone maintain weight who isn't into a sufficient amount of exercise.

If the prescribing of a maintenance diet doesn't work, the prescribing of an exercise program does. There is no accurate way to measure exactly how much exercise the average person needs, but I believe that in the majority of my patients, burning up an extra 400 to 500 calories a day above and beyond their normal activities will go a long way toward keeping them thin. This applies to those who have no metabolic problem whatsoever as well as those I'm treating for hypothyroidism. Of course, the latter group must be taking the proper dose of thyroid hormone or even that 400 to 500 calories of hard work will not maintain them.

How is this accomplished? With cardiovascular (aerobic) exercise. I don't favor one type over another. Your personal preferences should dictate this, but you must burn up 500 calories a day and you shouldn't miss more than one or two days a week. Many of my patients are members of well-equipped exercise facilities, and they can accomplish burning 500 calories per day at those places. Whether they choose the treadmill, the stepping machines, the ski machines, or the bicycles or a combination of several of them isn't as important as whether they are consistent.

There is a tendency for these places to advocate weight training at the expense of cardiovascular exercise, and I think you should be alert to that. Many of these "personal trainers" with the beautiful bodies can make a strong case for weight lifting. I don't see the necessity for it and I think it can actually be counterproductive, particularly if the time spent on the weights (or the weight machines) is borrowed from the time on the aerobic activity. The only real argument for weight training, in my opinion, comes from studies that seem to suggest it reduces the development of osteoporosis in women. I don't know if anyone has compared weight training with straight cardiovascular exercise as to that benefit.

It is difficult to assign calorie values per minute or per hour to various activities. This is particularly true when it comes to machines, which can be quite variable in the amount of effort required to work on them correctly. Many of the machines come with caloric expenditure readouts, and although I don't have much confidence in these calculations, they can still serve as a guide. They are certainly better than working totally in the dark. If you belong to an exercise facility, ask for their help in determining what you must do to burn up 500 calories.

The simplest activity is walking. It requires the least amount of preparation and you don't have to purchase designer tights to do it, nor does it require a paid membership. The streets for the moment are still free for you to use. You must walk at the right pace or you're wasting your time and not accomplishing the goal. The pace is fifteen minutes (or faster) for each mile covered. That's fast walking, possibly as fast as you can walk. If you were to cover your mile in much less time, you wouldn't be walking, you would be jogging or running. That too would be acceptable. There are arguments in favor of walking over jogging, and vice versa, and you must decide what is right for you. Just remember the 500 calories.

You must have asked yourself by now, When is he going to mention the diet for maintenance? The answer is now, except that there is none. I've already told you that the biggest failure in the whole weight-loss scenario is failure of most people to maintain the weight they have achieved. This is in spite of all the well-meaning efforts of those who have provided such well-thought-out maintenance diets. I no longer waste paper supplying these, and I don't waste my breath advocating them. I know that the odds of my patient staying on the diet, particularly if she doesn't have to stare me in the face periodically, are nil. The key is exercise, constantly, and enough of it, and in the majority of cases that will do it. Remember, you must first achieve your proper weight.

Since I don't supply a diet and in fact declare that there is no diet, does that mean you can eat everything your little heart desires? In my own practice I generally say yes, but sadly add before the end of the sentence, "within reason." That is, of course, the catch. What is within reason for one isn't within reason for another. So this is where you will have to feel your way. I've found that the vast majority of those with normal thyroid function, or with thyroid function that has been brought up to normal with medication, will maintain their weight eating very comfortably as long as they burn up the required calories. For most this can mean a dessert after dinner a few times a week, a daily glass of wine with the meal, and popcorn at the movies. There are areas where overdosing can catch up with you—things like regular sodas, sugar in coffee, etc. Why not continue to drink diet sodas and use artificial sweetener?

Of course you aren't limited to 500 calories' worth of exercise a day. If you've become a fanatic, as some do, you may do more. That will give you even more leeway when it comes to food. Bear in mind that each of you is different. What works for one doesn't necessarily work for another. Experiment to see how much exercise you need for your particular eating preferences. It may not be much fun maintaining weight, but it is certainly a nicer task to contemplate than losing weight.

As for your thyroid, if it was determined that there is simply not a problem there, what I've just given you is your method. If, however, you're one of those who has been shown to burn calories insufficiently and you've been put on thyroid hormone by your doctor, you must be vigilant to see that the amount you're getting is proper. The chances are that you feel much better after taking the thyroid hormone than you did before. You can use this general feeling as a benchmark of how you should feel in the future. Your requirement for thyroid hormone could change over time. You should be vigilant to look for this possibility. In some ways you're more qualified to suspect that a change is necessary than your doctor. You're the one who knows how you feel. Be assertive with him, but not obnoxious. You must preserve the relationship.

On a number of occasions I have had to raise the daily dose of thyroid hormone in a patient. I've also had to lower it, but much less frequently. Even in those cases, I don't think it was because of a true change in metabolism, but rather simply a matter of having prescribed a larger dose than was necessary.

As a parting word, I would like you to know that I've sincerely given you the information that has come from my years of dealing with overweight patients, with emphasis on those with hypothyroidism. I know other doctors may disagree. I suspect that most of that disagreement will come from those who strictly follow the literature rather than relying on their own hands-on experience. A lot of people in my own medical practice have been helped by taking my advice. I hope this advice will help you.

I would welcome hearing from you. My Web page awaits you. Contact me at www.drsiegal.com.

Summing Up

- Methods advocated for maintaining weight that concentrate on lifetime eating habits are notable failures because the public refuses to adhere to them.
- For the achieved weight to be maintained, the subject must have reached a proper goal weight.
- Weight maintenance is best accomplished by using exercise as the means rather than diet.

Appendix A: Prescribing Thyroid Hormone When the Gland Is Normal

A definition of euthyroid is a good place to start. This is a medical term that refers to a thyroid gland that functions normally—that is to say, one that supplies the right amount of thyroid hormone, neither too much nor too little.

By now, you're aware that I question the common way "too much" or "too little" is determined. The majority of doctors will look at the results of laboratory blood tests, often only one, the TSH test, and make the determination. The fact that I disagree with this method doesn't negate my acceptance of the definition in the previous paragraph. The hallmark of hypothyroidism is "too little," and I've already explored in detail how I determine "too little."

The question arises, Might the use of prescribed thyroid hormone have any place as a medication for those who are euthyroid, those with normal thyroid function? Earlier in the book I've emphatically stated that I have no experience with doing this. I've confined my prescribing of thyroid hormone to those whom I've diagnosed as having hypothyroidism. Perhaps I should have underlined that previous sentence, since I would not want to have my mention of thyroid hormone for the euthyroid misconstrued. *At this time, I don't advocate the use of thyroid hormone as a medication for those who are euthyroid.* I italicized the last statement to give it emphasis, and don't be surprised if you see it repeated more than once in the pages to follow.

Is there a case for prescribing it? No, but there may be in the future. I cannot make a case for prescribing thyroid to people with normal thyroid glands but I can certainly make a case for extensive study of its effect on euthyroid individuals in order to determine if it has value in those people. The effect of using thyroid hormone in some patients is so dramatic that it seems to fulfill its being designated a wonder drug. Of course, I'm speaking of the use of natural thyroid hormone, which, as you know, is my preference. To simplify this section, I will not differentiate among the specific hormonal products, but will lump them together as "thyroid hormone" or simply "thyroid." Yes, I can make a strong case for finding out if it can benefit those who don't have hypothyroidism.

Given that the differences in the varying degrees of hypothyroidism are so subtle, it is easy to see that it may be difficult to draw a fine line between those who have a minimal case, the so-called subclinical variety, and those who have nothing more than a suspicious symptom or two. Could someone in this category feel better by taking an even smaller dose of thyroid than I usually prescribe? The standard smallest tablet of natural thyroid available is about 15 milligrams. Might 7.5 milligrams or even a smaller amount have some value?

I will have no difficulty finding doctors who reject this idea. They will undoubtedly take the position that the hormone is specific for replacement in those who are shown to have a deficiency and could be harmful to anyone else. If they were pressed to explain how thyroid hormone could be harmful, I would expect to hear that it is known to raise blood pressure and pulse rate. One who doesn't need it might become jittery or shaky. It could cause palpitations. I will be the first to concur that those are all possibilities. I would then ask these dissenters if they've ever prescribed a medication that had that same potential for adverse effects upon a patient. Did they do it with the hope that it would help even though there was a chance of an adverse effect? Let's look at a concrete example.

I think it is common for doctors, when confronted with a patient who has a runny nose or is sneezing, to prescribe medications that contain drugs such as phenylephrine, phenylpropanolamine, or pseudoephedrine. I realize that those words are a mouthful, but they are all substances in the category of vasoconstrictors—they narrow blood vessels. In the process of doing so, they tend to shrink the membranes that line the nasal passages, and thus facilitate the passage of air into the nose. These types of medications are prescribed universally and can even be purchased without a prescription in the form of various "cold" preparations or allergy treatments. They are commonly referred to as decongestants.

One characteristic of these decongestants is that they have the common side effect of increasing the pulse rate and elevating the blood pressure. There are even dire warnings that the doctor or the purchaser must use caution when the user has certain medical conditions. I wonder if the doctor who prescribes these for the patient who has a moderately fast pulse or a blood pressure approaching borderline exerts as much caution as he might advocate for trying thyroid on a patient who could benefit from thyroid medication.

The fact is that such a prejudice toward the use of thyroid in all but the most blatant cases is so prevalent that doctors don't apply the same set of rules to it as they do to decongestants. I might speculate that using decongestants in the wrong patient is far more dangerous than using thyroid in the wrong patient.

I might get an argument as to the wisdom of my last statement. If so, I would challenge anyone to do a better search of the literature than I've done and demonstrate proof that the trial of thyroid in a supposed euthyroid individual carries more danger than, let us say, prescribing aspirin to someone who has never taken the drug before.

Aspirin has occasionally been referred to as the wonder drug of the century. I would guess that it has taken away more headaches than any other drug in history. Many arthritis sufferers rely on it to quell their agony. It is now the first medicine to be given with a suspected heart attack. In spite of these wondrous testimonials, aspirin can also be very dangerous. It has been implicated in precipitating Reye's syndrome in children. Many people owe their ulcers to using aspirin, and it could be life-threatening to someone allergic to it.

We don't generally hold back on prescribing medications that have great potential to heal and only minimal potential to cause harm to the subject. We must factor into the equation whether any harm done is reversible. Can it be stopped in its tracks? When a doctor observes an uncomfortably fast pulse in someone who has taken a decongestant, he simply stops the use of the decongestant. If our patient breaks out in a rash after his first aspirin tablet, we discontinue it and mark on his chart, "Allergic to aspirin." Could not thyroid medication be stopped at the first sign of a problem?

This might sound like I'm advocating the use of thyroid in the euthyroid. *I'm certainly not.* It's time for repetition. *At this time, I don't advocate the use of thyroid hormone as a medication for those who are euthyroid.* Is there a time when I will? Possibly. When its use in that area has been carefully studied and the potential for benefit far outweighs the potential for harm.

Do I see this happening in the future? Quite possibly. There is certainly a case for investigating that possibility. It may be that much smaller doses than are customary can benefit the euthyroid. There may be those who have some elements of hypothyroidism that my MFI test doesn't pick up. But for the present, don't even think of trying to talk your doctor into prescribing thyroid if you aren't hypothyroid.

And once again: *At this time, I don't advocate the use of thyroid hormone as a medication for those who are euthyroid.*

Appendix B: Historical Perspectives on Eating Meat and Fat

We should well ask ourselves why we love meat and fat so much. Like many other characteristics we possess, the answer probably lies in our genes. We, the human race, are meat and fat eaters because our ancestors were meat and fat eaters.

I see my share of vegetarians. They are apt to point out that we humans have more of the physical characteristics of other primates like chimps or gorillas, essentially vegetarian animals. They point to the teeth and the fingernails and the thumbs, etc. They say we don't have the same kind of teeth as lions and tigers or even the family dog. I can't argue with that. It really doesn't look like we were designed for meat-eating. But what we were designed for and what serves us best aren't necessarily the same.

The process of evolution changes us so that we can adapt from what we were designed for. Were we designed to travel in steel vehicles with rubber tires, to leave them in underground parking garages while we go to work in an office on the fiftieth floor of a skyscraper? We may not have been designed to eat other animals, but that's exactly what we've been doing ever since we got up off all fours.

Early man was clearly a hunter-gatherer. He hunted animals and gathered fruits, nuts, and berries. Every evidence is that the hunting was more productive than the gathering. It takes a lot of berries to satisfy the needs of an extended family, but a wild boar all by itself can do the job admirably. And the fatter it was, the more food energy (calories) it provided. Early man wasn't interested in how his cholesterol was doing. He wanted the most calories he could get for his "buck." For over a million years, man has been a hunter and a meat-eater. He wasn't able to go to the supermarket and pick out fresh fruits and vegetables.

The nice thing about we humans is that we do adapt. Adaptation isn't limited to humans. All species adapt. If you eat meat long enough because it is expedient to do so, even though you were originally designed for other things, your body undergoes changes. Over a million years this adaptation becomes more established, until eventually you fare better in the new environment than in the old.

Over virtually all of man's history, the quest for food was his chief occupation. His day was spent searching for food. Man had to go where the food was. He was for the most part nomadic. He followed the herd, so to speak. The plant foods he ate were gathered. You can't grow your own crops if you're constantly on the move. He was a hunter. A number of anthropological writers have said that the predatory predilection survives today. We're still essentially hunters; it is instinctual.

One of the better authors on this subject was Robert Ardrey. He was actually a writer of plays as well as Hollywood films. But his true love was anthropology and ethology, and he devoted years to research in this field. Between 1961 and 1976 Mr. Ardrey wrote four books on the subject of the origins of man's basic nature. He talked with the foremost researchers of his time. Ardrey gives the impression of, at the same time, both loving and hating the human race. His first book, *African Genesis,* was sort of a homage to Raymond Dart, who made a most important discovery, the bones of a man who lived 4 to 5 million years ago in Africa, and whom Dart named *Australopithecus africanus.*

Dart was convinced that his *Australopithecus* was both a tool maker and big-game hunter. His find broke new ground, for it moved man's origins from Asia to Africa, and emphasized our hunting nature. His paper that followed, *The Predatory Nature of Man,* wasn't well received. It rocked the boat. Only most recently have his findings become more widely accepted.

By the time Robert Ardrey had written his fourth book, *The Hunting Hypothesis,* he seemed to have clearly developed his thesis:

> Man is man, and not a chimpanzee, because for millions
> upon millions of evolving years we killed for a living.

Ardrey knew that for perhaps 500,000 years, our ancestors were continuously dependent upon killing to survive. Because of our "big brain" and our inventive nature, we were able to do it well, perhaps surpassing all other animals in that skill.

Not everyone agreed, but Ardrey had the evidence, and his proof was hard to refute. His critics were armed more with rhetoric than with solid evidence. His friend Louis Leakey, possibly the most famous researcher in anthropology of the time, wasn't as certain as Ardrey that man had been such a great hunter. There was no dispute that man was a carnivore, a meat-eater, but Leakey leaned toward the notion that man got his meat by settling for "roadkill," or by being a scavenger. In other words he felt that early man was more inclined to let other animals do his dirty work, the kill, and that he simply took the leftovers.

Ardrey disagreed. He didn't believe man could sustain life that way. He felt that if man had the guts to steal food from fierce beasts, he had the courage to go after his own prey. In a debate with Louis Leakey, reprinted in *Psychology Today* in 1972, Ardrey makes his point:

If we go back 500,000 years to *Homo sapiens,* the big-brained man, there isn't much question about what went on. They were definitely hunters. This heritage has had a tremendous effect upon us in terms of natural selection. Those men who had an efficient capacity for violence, who enjoyed violence, were the men who survived and passed on their genes. If you didn't like to go out and hunt, you wouldn't get the girl, and you wouldn't get any food—you'd just be an extra mouth to feed. And I would assert that we didn't live off of spinach. This is a fashionable point of view much promoted in American anthropology. Lettuce is great for diets, but not for men who have to work for a living. We had to live off meat.

Dr. Lyall Watson independently developed similar ideas, but with some differences. Watson, a South African zoologist and a director of the Johannesburg Zoo, shared Ardrey's opinion of the killing nature of early man. In his book *The Omnivorous Ape,* he states:

Man is what he is and does what he does because he once was a killer. He was hungry and needed food, and the food he most wanted was meat. So he applied his growing brain to the problem of killing—and started a chain of circumstances that still affects our lives today. Because our ancestors needed greater speed, they became more upright and today we have vertical men. Because they needed artificial weapons, tools were developed and today we have elaborate instrumentation. Because cooperation was essential, their brains became even more complex, and a language and a culture came into being. Today we also have spinal disorders, ballistic missiles and racial disturbances, but we have had to take the bad with the good. Both were produced by our diet.

Notice that Watson at least seems to be saying that man "was" a killer. He uses the past tense. That should make a lot of people a lot more comfortable. He obviously differs from Ardrey in that he believes we have channeled that aggressive nature in more socially acceptable directions.

> Man relinquished his role as a killer and hunter when he became a settled farmer about 10,000 years ago. He became domesticated and well fed, but he still needed to hunt. . . . In a million years of hunting, man formed close ties with other adult males in the tribe and grew used to a life involving constant risks and challenges. So he turned work into an activity that involved him, with other men, in a recurring gamble that has many characteristics of the hunt. To take an example from only one kind of work, he set aside hunting grounds (business centers) where the prey (his rivals) could be stalked (with the aid of industrial espionage) and captured (in a take-over bid). In the all-male gatherings that have always followed the hunt, the money hunter is able to boast his prowess and of the "killing" he has just made.

It wasn't until about 10,000 years ago that things began to change. Most authorities put man's entry into farming at between 8,000 and 13,000 years ago. Things moved very slowly back then. A hundred generations would go by and there was possibly no change in the farming techniques. Some experts feel that although man farmed, he really didn't get his act together until about 5,000 years ago.

Desmond Morris, another zoologist, took note of this in his entertaining and informative best-seller of the late sixties, *The Naked Ape:*

> We were driven to become flesh-eaters only by environmental circumstances, and now that we have the environment under control, with elaborately cultivated

crops at our disposal, we might be expected to return to
our ancient primate feeding patterns. In essence, this is
the vegetarian . . . creed, but it has had remarkably little success. The urge to eat meat appears to have become
too deep-seated. Given the opportunity to devour flesh,
we are loth to relinquish the pattern.

According to Watson, you're thus unique in the animal world.
He recognizes four eating patterns: insectivores, herbivores
(plant-eaters), carnivores (flesh-eaters), and omnivores (eaters of a
mixed diet). Many animals have undergone evolutionary changes
in their diets. Some have made only a single change during their
history. Others have made two changes. Man is the only animal
to make three such changes.

The only animal ever to move from insect eating to fruit
picking to meat eating to eating absolutely anything.
Man.

Of course, we men lack some of the characteristics necessary to
really do a good job of digesting plant foods. It's not surprising.
We've just started to eat them. We are, so to speak, trying them
out. Cows, for example, are real herbivores. They digest the cellulose that makes up the main portion of fruits and vegetables.
We, on the other hand, can't digest cellulose, so it passes right
through us. That isn't necessarily bad. Many writers (including
this one) have written books extolling the virtues of eating this fibrous material. It apparently acts as somewhat of a sweeping
compound to cleanse the intestinal tract.

The dawn of agriculture required our hunters to stay put and
watch the crops grow. This was a major change, and it was the
major force in the growth of villages, cities, countries, and
boundary lines. Agriculture changed the human experience and
we now added plant foods to our diets.

In the scheme of things, 10,000 years is an instant. It is an in-
significant period of time for an adaptation to take place in the

human race. It is unlikely that we're physically much different from our 10,000-year-old ancestors.

Evolutionary changes take place slowly, very slowly. I cannot emphasize enough how slow the process is. We commonly describe things using the adjective *slow*. We may speak of our trip home from work as being slow, or say that Congress is slow to act, or that Third World countries are slowly becoming industrialized. Believe me, those are all fast. Evolution is slow.

Human beings haven't changed much in the last few thousand years. Borrow a dozen men from one of Caesar's legions, put shorts and Nikes on them and send them to your local fitness club, and they will get lost among all the other bodies. Or put the right suit on one of them, give him a good haircut, and let him walk down Madison Avenue with an attaché case and no one will notice anything unusual.

As for our nutritional needs, we're probably still cavemen. That's why we still love meat. That's why the fast-food restaurants. That's why the steak houses. That's why the cookouts.

That is one of the reasons I prefer a high-protein diet for my patients. They also prefer it and that is important, because if they aren't repelled by the food selections, they are more inclined to stay with the diet. A more important reason for my preference is because a high-protein diet works.

Appendix C: How to Customize Your Diet Test

The MFI test I described earlier is the one I recommend. It results in a twofold benefit. Not only do you learn whether your thyroid is causing your weight problems, but you also lose a substantial amount of weight in the process.

There will be those of you who have had a lot of experience with past diets, and there will be others who have never dieted seriously. For some, 1,000 calories a day may be a fearful prospect. I know from experience that it isn't. You can do it. The expectation of spending the rest of your days wearing normal-sized clothing should spur you on. Nonetheless, I'll give you an alternative.

There is nothing magic about a 1,000-calorie diet. I could calculate valid results on my patients while they were eating any number of calories per day. I could even arrive at the result if they ate a widely different number of calories from day to day. In order for me to do so, there really are only two things I need to know. *I must know how many calories my subject consumed for the entire twenty-eight-day period, and I must know exactly how much weight was lost during that time.* Once I have that information, the rest is the kind of thing we do every day with our pocket calculators.

Why did I not present this information earlier? I've already told you. I believe that if 1,000 calories is chosen and the subject adheres to my food choices in accomplishing it, hunger will be minimal, there will be impressive weight loss, and there may be no need for the pocket calculator. By standardizing to 1,000 calories, I was able to make the whole thing very simple for you to accomplish. I did all the calculations in advance and gave you nice neat little tables to work with. Were I to have allowed variable amounts of calories, I would have had to supply you with a similar set of tables for each different calorie count. That would have been quite complex, and there would have been too much room for error.

For the adventurous willing to make their own calculations, I present the following method. Get your thinking cap on.

One of the two bits of information you need is easy. Weigh yourself at the beginning of the twenty-eight days and also at the end, just as specified earlier in the book. You need to know how many pounds you lost eating a certain number of calories. The "certain number of calories" is going to take dedication.

You're going to count every calorie you ate during the entire twenty-eight-day period meticulously and mark them down. It sounds more difficult than it is. You're obviously embarking on this alternate method because you're going to follow a diet other than the one I recommend. That's okay. In a sense, the original diet also required counting the calories, but the idea was to shoot for 1,000, and if you varied a bit, you kept a record of how many you went over 1,000 on an Excess Calorie Sheet. If you're going to follow Test B (Do you like that name?), then you will do exactly the same thing, except the excess calories are presumably going to be greater. What you will be marking down on your Excess Calorie Sheet will be bigger numbers such as "460" or "530" instead of perhaps "175" or "80." If you aren't going to be marking down numbers that large, there is little reason for you to be following Test B. You are back to Dr. Siegal's original test diet.

In Chapter 13 you were asked to calculate your uncorrected caloric maintenance level based on a 1,000-calorie diet. What is accomplished by this is that you learn your daily maintenance level after you've spent four weeks eating *exactly* 1,000 calories per day. The UCML table is still appropriate because, in a sense, you're still basing your performance on 1,000 calories per day, but you're simply exceeding your quota by a much larger amount than I advised. However, you can't use the table titled CCML because the number of calories in excess is now "off the charts," as they say. One solution is to make your own chart. Don't panic. You don't really have to make a chart, but you do have to make some calculations.

Here are your complete instructions:

Use the MFI Calculation Form on page 161.

1. Write in your weight on Day 1.
2. Write in your weight on Day 29.
3. Subtract Line (2) from Line (1).
4. Obtain your UCML from the UCML Table on page 164.
5. Write in your excess calories for the entire twenty-eight days on Line (5).
6. Divide that number by 28 and jot it down somewhere as the value of your daily excess (DE). Add the UCML to the DE. This is your CCML.
7. Get your BBW in Line (7) from the BBW Table on page 166.
8. Choose the proper SCML Table on pages 168–171 and write in your SCML.
9. Divide the CCML in Line (6) by the SCML in Line (8). Move the decimal point two digits to the right and round it off to the nearest whole number. That is your MFI.

This example illustrates the process. Here is the MFI Calculation Form:

MFI Calculation Form

Metabolic Function Index

(1) **Day 1 Date** *9/4/99* **Weight (nude)**
(Early morning)

| 186 |

(2) **Day 29 Date** *10/3/99* **Weight (nude)**
(Early morning)

| 184 |

(3) **28-day weight loss**
Subtract line (2) from line (1).

| 2 |

(4) **UCML (Uncorrected Caloric Maintenance Level)**
From the UCML Table on page 164.

| 1,250 |

(5) **EC (Total Excess Calories for the 28 Days)**
From your own list of excess calories for the entire 28 days.

| 11,760 |

(6) **CCML (Corrected Caloric Maintenance Level)**
See the Excess Calories Table on page 165.

| 1,670 |

(7) **BBW (Baseline Body Weight)**
See BBW Table on page 166.

| 149 |

(8) **SCML (Standard Caloric Maintenance Level)**
See the proper SCML Table for your sex, age group, and activity level
on pages 168–171. Use the BBW in (7) above to determine your SCML.

| 2,275 |

(9) **Metabolic Function Index (MFI)**
Divide line (6) by line (8). Move the decimal point
2 digits to the right.

| *73*% |

The subject is a thirty-eight-year-old female who is five feet eight inches tall and who has a large frame. She is rated as moderately active. The only difference from the usual way of calculating her MFI as explained in Chapter 13 is when it comes to the CCML.

The DE was calculated by dividing her total excess for the month in Line (5) by 28. Then in Line (6), add the UCML to the DE. This total becomes your CCML. The rest of the task is the same as explained in Chapter 13.

You may now go back to Chapter 13 for an interpretation of the results.

Appendix D: Determining Your Frame Size

When considering such subjects as ideal or normal weight, it is customary to classify individuals by the size of their body "frames." Generally, the classifications are small, medium, and large frames.

Although it isn't difficult for any of us to judge someone's frame size by our own past experience, it is desirable to have some objective standard upon which to rely. One such standard involves taking a measurement across the elbow. The distance between the bony protrusions on the two sides of the elbow is measured.

The process is easier if you get someone to help in the procedure.

How to Measure Your Frame Size

1. Locate the two prominent bones that extend outward on each side of your elbow at the ends of your elbow crease.
2. Place a letter-sized sheet of paper on a flat tabletop.

3. Center your elbow on the sheet of paper with your arm straight, elbow crease and palm up.

4. With a sharp pencil, accurately mark the position of each of these bones on the paper so that the distance between the two marks measures the distance across your elbow. Be sure to keep the pencil vertical.

5. With a ruler, measure the distance between the two pencil marks.

6. Use the table below to determine your frame size based on your sex and age.

ELBOW MEASUREMENT

Age	Small	Medium	Large
Males			
18–24	≤2⅝"	>2⅝" and <3¹⁄₁₆"	≥3¹⁄₁₆"
25–34	≤2⅝"	>2⅝" and <3⅛"	≥3⅛"
35–44	≤2⅝"	>2⅝" and <3³⁄₁₆"	≥3³⁄₁₆"
45–54	≤2⅝"	>2⅝" and <3³⁄₁₆"	≥3³⁄₁₆"
55–64	≤2⅝"	>2⅝" and <3³⁄₁₆"	≥3³⁄₁₆"
65–74	≤2⅝"	>2⅝" and <3³⁄₁₆"	≥3³⁄₁₆"
Females			
18–24	≤2¼"	>2¼" and <2⁹⁄₁₆"	≥2⁹⁄₁₆"
25–34	≤2¼"	>2¼" and <2¹¹⁄₁₆"	≥2¹¹⁄₁₆"
35–44	≤2¼"	>2¼" and <2¹³⁄₁₆"	≥2¹³⁄₁₆"
45–54	≤2¼"	>2¼" and <2⅞"	≥2⅞"
55–64	≤2⁵⁄₁₆"	>2⁵⁄₁₆" and <2⅞"	≥2⅞"
65–74	≤2⁵⁄₁₆"	>2⁵⁄₁₆" and <2⅞"	≥2⅞"

Example: *A forty-year-old female with a measurement of 2½" has a medium frame.*

Appendix E: Evaluating Your Activity Level

In Chapter 13, in the process of calculating your Metabolic Function Index, you are asked to evaluate your activity level. You are given three choices: sedentary, moderate, and active. If you were simply to make the choice without serious study of your activities, I think you would probably guess right. Yet I have seen patients who were not even close in their estimation of their activity levels.

A worker in a busy office might tell me, "My job is so active that I don't have a minute's rest. Yes, I sit, but a million times a day I have to get up and run to another desk and then run back to answer a phone call. By the end of the day, I'm beat." I may risk bursting her bubble, but I need to pry for more information. I try to pin her down to a more realistic number than "a million times." I suggest numbers. Between this and that number? Eventually, I get an admission that seems reasonable. Let's settle on twenty-five, which is probably overestimating.

This lady sits for most of the day. Each excursion to another desk takes perhaps one minute. Does she really run, or is that a figure of speech? When she gets to her destination does she stand still and talk for a while? What is the bottom line? I will give her, at best, a total of thirty minutes of ordinary walking and the rest of the time sitting at a desk. I dare say, her day doesn't even compare with an ordinary shopping trip to the mall. It just seems to her that she is getting a lot of exercise. Clearly, she is sedentary.

Don't give such sports as golf or bowling more credit than they deserve. I've had to disparage the exercise value of bowling to too many patients. Let's look at the facts.

If you are a particularly bad bowler, you will roll 20 balls per game. If we analyze that activity and put a time line on it, we will have the following:

1. Getting up from the bench and picking up the ball—5 seconds.
2. Holding the ball and staring at the pins—5 seconds.
3. Pulling your arm back, taking three steps, bending your knees, and releasing the ball—4 seconds.
4. Staring at the result—3 seconds.
5. After every other ball, walking back to your seat—5 seconds.

It looks like the whole process took about 20 seconds, though only 4 of those involved anything more than walking or standing. That means that for each game the bad bowler has 3 minutes or so of total *activity* (I can't bring myself to use the word *exercise*), but really only 80 seconds of that even resembles exercise. Now multiply those figures by the number of games.

I hope you see the point. It is easy to delude ourselves into believing that we are more active than we really are. I rarely see anyone err on the opposite side—that is, underestimate their activity level.

As for golf, it's really not much better. If you walk the course, it's a nice walk, but you stand still more than you walk. If you use a cart, forget it. Try adding up the number of seconds spent swinging the clubs. Putting certainly shouldn't count. I know I'm going to be hearing from golfers on this one.

It's quite important that you select the proper activity level. At the extreme ends, a mistake could account for a thousand calories or more per day. An area for confusion arises when there is a mixture of varied activities. What about the guy who sits at a desk five days a week but runs six miles both on Saturday and Sunday? There are people who do just that.

Your principal daily activity is not hard to evaluate. If you sit at a desk or drive a car most of the day, that is considered sedentary. (Brain work burns up very few calories.) If you are on the move constantly and virtually never sit down (standing still excluded), you may be in the moderate class. If you never put down your shovel, you are active.

Let's use as a rule of thumb that a sedentary individual who burns an extra 2,000 calories per week in more energetic activity moves to the moderate class. One with moderate activity has to burn an extra 4,000 a week to get into the active class. "Active" is not achieved easily. Some pretty good guesses have been made when it comes to estimating how many calories various activities burn up per hour. Let's look at what some activities are worth in terms of calories.

Walking, brisk	300–400
Bicycling, fast	300–400
Gardening	300–375
Weight training	150–350
Housework	150–200
Calisthenics	300–400
Tennis	400–550

These are only examples of various activities, and you can interpolate them into other activities. It is impossible to assign absolutely dependable calorie counts for each activity because there is such variation in how they are performed, as well as in the weight of the person involved in them. Estimate to the best of your ability.

> **Example:** *You have a sedentary occupation but you play two hours of tennis (singles) twice a week. You are probably burning an extra 2,000 calories a week and therefore you would move up into the moderate category.*

Exercise machines at many gyms frequently give a readout of calories consumed. I don't have much confidence in their absolute accuracy, but they are probably better than your own guessing. Use them.

Appendix F: Bibliography

Barnes, B. O., "On the Genesis of Atherosclerosis," *Journal of the American Geriatrics Society,* 21(8): 350–354.

Barnes, B., "Basal Temperature versus Basal Metabolism," *Journal of the American Medical Association,* 119(14): 1072–1074.

Billewicz, W. Z.; Chapman, R. S.; Crooks, J.; Day, M. E.; Gossage, J.; Wayne, S. E.; & Young, J. A., "Statistical Methods Applied to the Diagnosis of Hypothyroidism," *Quarterly Journal of Medicine,* 38(150): 255–266.

Bishnoi, A., & Sachmechi, I., "Thyroid Disease During Pregnancy," *American Family Physician,* 53(1): 215–220.

Boothby, W., & Sandiford, I., "Summary of the Basal Metabolism Data on 8,614 Subjects with Especial Reference to the Normal Standards for the Estimation of the Basal Metabolic Rate," *The Journal of Biological Chemistry,* 54(4): 783–803.

Bradfield, R. B., & Jourdan, M. H., "Relative Importance of Specific Dynamic Action in Weight-Reduction Diets," *The Lancet,* 2(7830): 640–643.

Briefel, R. R.; McDowell, M. A.; Alaimo, K.; Caughman, C. R.; Bischof, M. D.; & Johnson, C. L., "Total Energy Intake of the U.S. Population: The Third National Health and Nutrition Examination Survey, 1988–1991," *The American Journal of Clinical Nutrition,* 62: 1072S–1080S.

Bunevicius, R.; Kazanavicius, G.; Zalinkevicius, R.; & Pragne, A. J., "Effects of Thyroxine as Compared with Thyroxine Plus Triiodothyronine in Patients with Hypothyroidism," *The New England Journal of Medicine,* 340(6): 424–429.

Butte, N. F.; Moon, J. K.; Wong, W. W.; Hopkins, J. M.; & Smith, E. O'Brian, "Energy Requirements from Infancy to Adulthood," *The American Journal of Clinical Nutrition,* 62: 1047S–1052S.

Calloway, D. H., & Zanni, E., "Energy Requirements and Energy Expenditure of Elderly Men," *The American Journal of Clinical Nutrition,* 33: 2088–2092.

Campbell, R. C.; Welle, S. L.; & Seaton, T. B., "Specific Dynamic Action Revisited: Studies of Hormonal Regulation of Energy Expenditure in Man," *Transactions of the American Clinical and Climatological Association,* 99: 136–143.

Cheraskin, E., "A Different Methodologic Approach to 'Ideal Weight': A Study of the Ponderal Index (PI)," *Medical Hypothesis,* 29: 55–58.

Clark, H. D., & Hoffer, J. L., "Reappraisal of the Resting Metabolic Rate of Normal Young Men," *The American Journal of Clinical Nutrition,* 53: 21–26.

Cushing, G. W., "Subclinical Hypothyroidism: Understanding Is the Key to Decision Making," *Postgraduate Medicine,* 94(1): 95–107.

Denicoff, K. D.; Joffe, R. T.; Lakshmanan, M. C.; Robbins, J.; & Rubinow, D. R., "Neuropsychiatric Manifestations of Altered Thyroid State," *American Journal of Psychiatry,* 147: 94–99.

Doucet, J.; Trivalle, C.; Chassagne, P.; Perol, M. B.; Vuillermet, P.; Manchon, N. D.; Menard, J. F.; & Bercoff, E., "Does Age Play a Role in Clinical Presentation of Hypothyroidism?" *Journal of the American Geriatrics Society,* 42(9): 984–986.

Drinka, P. J., & Nolten, W. E., "Subclinical Hypothyroidism in the Elderly: To Treat or Not to Treat?" *The American Journal of the Medical Sciences,* 295(2): 125–128.

Faulkner, R. A., & Bailey, D. A., "Critical Evaluation of Frame Size Determination in the 1983 Metropolitan Life Weight for Height Tables," *Canadian Journal of Public Health,* 80: 369–372.

Feldmesser-Reiss, E. E., "The Application of Triiodothyronine in the Treatment of Mental Disorders," *Journal of Nervous and Mental Disease,* 127: 540–546.

Feurer, I. D.; Crosby, L. O.; Buzby, G. P.; Rosato, E. F.; & Mullen, J. L., "Resting Energy Expenditure in Morbid Obesity," *Annals of Surgery,* 197(1): 17–21.

Flat, J. P., "Body Composition, Respiratory Quotient, and Weight Maintenance," *The American Journal of Clinical Nutrition,* 62: 1107S–1117S.

Frankenfield, D. C.; Muth, E. R.; & Rowe, W. A., "The Harris-Benedict Studies of Human Basal Metabolism: History and Limitations," *Journal of the American Dietetic Association,* 98(4): 439–445.

Friedman, M. I., "Control of Energy Intake by Energy Metabolism," *The American Journal of Clinical Nutrition,* 62: 1096S–1100S.

Frisancho, R., "New Standards of Weight and Body Composition by Frame Size and Height for Assessment of Nutritional Status of Adults and the Elderly," *The American Journal of Clinical Nutrition,* 40: 808–819.

Garrow, J. S., & Hawes, S. F., "The Role of Amino Acid Oxidation in Causing 'Specific Dynamic Action' in Man," *British Journal of Nutrition,* 27(1): 211–219.

Gold, M. S.; Pottash, A. L. C.; & Extein, I., "Hypothyroidism and Depression: Evidence from Complete Thyroid Function Evaluation," *JAMA,* 245(19): 1919–1922.

Gross, M. A., "Achilles-Reflex Timing in Diagnosis of Thyroid Status," *New York State Journal of Medicine,* 71(19): 2283–2291.

Gruhn, J. G.; Barsano, C. P.; & Kumar, Y., "The Development of Tests of Thyroid Function," *Archives of Pathology and Laboratory Medicine,* 111: 84–100.

Gupta, S. P.; Kimar, V.; & Ahuja, M. S., "Evaluation of Achilles Reflex Time as a Test of Thyroid Function," *Southern Medical Journal,* 66(7): 754–758.

Haggerty, J. J., Jr.; Stern, R. A.; Mason, G. A.; Beckwith, J.; Morey, C. E.; & Prange, A. J., Jr., "Subclinical Hypothyroidism: A Modifiable Risk Factor for Depression?" *American Journal of Psychiatry,* 150: 508–510.

Henley, W. N., & Koehnle, T. J., "Thyroid Hormones and the Treatment of Depression: An Examination of Basic Hormonal Actions in the Mature Mammalian Brain," *Synapse,* 27: 36–44.

Hernandez, J. J. C.; Garcia, J. M. M.; & Diez, L. C. G., "Primary Hypothyroidism and Human Spermatogenesis," *Archives of Andrology,* 25: 21–27.

Heymsfield, S. B.; Darby, P. C.; Muhlheim, L. S.; Gallagher, D.; Wolper, C.; & Allison, D. B., "The Calorie: Myth, Measurement, and Reality," *The American Journal of Clinical Nutrition,* 62: 1034S–1041S.

Hill, J. O.; Melby, C.; Johnson, S. L.; & Peters, J. C., "Physical Activity and Energy Requirements," *The American Journal of Clinical Nutrition,* 62: 1059S–1066S.

Himes, J. H., & Bouchard, C., "Do the New Metropolitan Life Insurance Weight-Height Tables Correctly Assess Body Frame and Body Fat Relationships?" *American Journal of Public Health,* 75(9): 1076–1079.

Howland, R. H., "Thyroid Dysfunction in Refractory Depression: Implications for Pathophysiology and Treatment," *Journal of Clinical Psychiatry,* 54: 47–54.

Ireton-Jones, C. S., & Turner, W. W., Jr., "Actual or Ideal Body Weight: Which Should Be Used to Predict Energy Expenditure?" *Journal of the American Dietetic Association,* 91(2): 193–195.

Jonckheer, M.; Block, P.; & Molter, F., "Use of the Achilles-Tendon Reflex in Thyroid Clinical Investigation," *Acta Endocrinologica,* 63(1): 175–184.

Klatsky, S. A., & Mason, P. N., "Thyroid Disorders Masquerading as Aging Changes," *Annals of Plastic Surgery,* 28(5): 420–426.

Klein, I., "Thyroid Hormone and the Cardiovascular System," *The American Journal of Medicine,* 88: 631–637.

Knapp, T. R., "A Methodological Critique of the 'Ideal Weight' Concept," *JAMA,* 250(4): 506–510.

Koutras, D. A., "Disturbances of Menstruation in Thyroid Disease," *Annals of the New York Academy of Sciences,* 816: 280–284.

Krebs, H. A., "The Cause of the Specific Dynamic Action of Foodstuffs," *Arzeneimittelforschung,* 10: 369–373.

Krupsky, M.; Flatau, E.; Yarom, R.; & Resnitzky, P., "Musculoskeletal Symptoms as a Presenting Sign of Long-standing Hypothyroidism," *Israel Journal of Medical Sciences,* 23: 1110–1113.

Krzanowski, J. J., "Thyroid Hormone: Basis for Its Hypocholesterolemic Effects," *Journal of the Florida Medical Association,* 78(6): 383–385.

Lindemann, C. G.; Zitrin, C. M.; & Klein, D. F., "Thyroid Dysfunction in Phobic Patients," *Journal of Clinical Psychiatry,* 54(2): 47–54.

Lusk, G., "The Fundamental Requirements of Energy for Proper Nutrition," *Journal of the American Medical Association,* 70(12): 821–824.

———, "The Physiological Effect of Undernutrition," *Physiological Reviews,* 1(4): 523–552.

Mariotti, S.; Barbesino, G.; Caturegli, P.; Bartalena, L.; Sansoni, P.; Fagnoni, F.; Monti, D.; Fagiolo, U.; Franceschi, C.; & Pinchera, A., "Complex Alteration of Thyroid Function in Healthy Centenarians," *Journal of Clinical Endocrinology and Metabolism,* 77(5): 1130–1134.

Matsuzawa, Y.; Tokunaga, K.; Kotani, K.; Keno, Y.; Kobayashi, T.; & Tarui, S., "Simple Estimation of Ideal Body Weight from Body Mass Index with the Lowest Morbidity," *Diabetes Research and Clinical Practice,* 10: S159–S164.

Mazzaferri, E. L., "Recognizing the Faces of Hypothyroidism," *Hospital Practice,* 93–110.

Mifflin, M. D.; St. Jeor, S. T.; Hill, L. A.; Scott, B. J.; Daugherty, S. A.; & Koh, Y. O., "A New Predictive Equation for Resting Energy Expenditure in Healthy Individuals," *The American Journal of Clinical Nutrition,* 51: 241–247.

Mitchell, H. H., "The Physiological Effects of Protein," *The Journal of Nutrition,* 1(3): 271–292.

Mitchell, M. C., "Comparison of Determinants of Frame Size in Older Adults," *Journal of the American Dietetic Association,* 93(1): 53–57.

Montoro, M.; Collea, J. V.; Frasier, S. D.; & Mestman, J. H., "Successful Outcome of Pregnancy in Women with Hypothyroidism," *Annals of Internal Medicine,* 94(1): 31–34.

Monzani, F.; del Guerra, P.; Caraccio, N.; Pruneti, C. A.; Pucci, E.; Luisi, M.; & Baschieri, L., "Subclinical Hypothyroidism: Neurobehavioral Features and Beneficial Effect of L-thyroxine Treatment," *Clinical Investigation,* 71: 367–371.

Mooney, C. J.; James, D. A.; & Kessenich, C. R., "Diagnosis and Management of Hypothyroidism in Pregnancy," *Journal of Obstetrical Gynecological Neonatal Nursing,* 27(4): 374–380.

Nordyke, R. A., & Gilbert, F. I., Jr., "The Achilles Reflex Thyroid Function Test: Evaluation of a New Instrument," *The American Journal of the Medical Sciences,* 259: 419–423.

Nuttall, F. Q., & Doe, R. P., "The Achilles Reflex in Thyroid Disorders," *Annals of Internal Medicine,* 61(2): 269–288.

Pavlou, K. N.; Hoefer, M. A.; & Blackburn, G. L., "Resting Energy Expenditure in Moderate Obesity: Predicting Velocity of Weight Loss," *Annals of Surgery,* 203(2): 136–141.

Powell, J. T.; Carter, G.; Woolcock, N.; Greenhalgh, R. M.; Fowler, P. B. S.; & Zadeh, J. A., "The Relationship Between Serum Cholesterol and Serum Thyrotropin in Women with Peripheral Arterial Disease," *Annals of Clinical Biochemistry,* 28: 316–319.

Rees-Jones, R. W., & Larsen, P. R., "Triiodothyronine and Thyroxine Content of Desiccated Thyroid Tablets," *Metabolism,* 26(11): 1213–1218.

Ridgway, E. C., "Modern Concepts of Primary Thyroid Gland Failure," *Clinical Chemistry,* 42(1): 179–182.

Roberts, S. B.; Fuss, P.; Heyman, M. B.; & Young, V. R., "Influence of Age on Energy Requirements," *The American Journal of Clinical Nutrition,* 62: 1053S–1058S.

Roza, M., & Shizgal, H. M., "The Harris-Benedict Equation Reevaluated: Resting Energy Requirements and the Body Cell Mass," *The American Journal of Clinical Nutrition,* 40: 168–182.

Santiago, G., & Kennedy, J., "On Specific Dynamic Action, Turnover, and Protein Synthesis," *Perspectives in Biology and Medicine,* 9(4): 578–585.

Sawin, C. T.; Hershman, J. M.; Fernandez-Garcia, R.; Ghazvinian, S.; Ganda, O. P.; & Azukizawa, M., "A Comparison of Thyroxine and Desiccated Thyroid in Patients with Primary Hypothyroidism," *Metabolism,* 27(10): 1518–1525.

Schneeberg, N. G., "Pseudo-hypothyroidism," *Postgraduate Medicine,* 79(7): 103–111.

Schultz, L. O., "Lose, Overweight, Desirable, Ideal: Where to Draw the Line in 1986?" *Journal of the American Dietetic Association,* 86(12): 1402–1407.

Seale, J. L., "Energy Expenditure Measurements in Relation to Energy Requirements," *The American Journal of Clinical Nutrition,* 62: 1042S–1046S.

Selenkow, H. A., "Hypothyroid Women with Rising Serum Cholesterol Values," *Consultant,* 26.

Shafer, R. B., & Nuttall, F. Q., "Achilles Reflex in Thyroid Disorders: A 10-year Clinical Evaluation," *The American Journal of the Medical Sciences,* 264(4): 313–317.

Souetre, E.; Salvati, E.; Wehr, T. A.; Sack, D. A.; Krebs, B.; & Darcourt, G., "Twenty-Four-Hour Profiles of Body Temperature and Plasma TSH in Bipolar Patients During Depression and During Remission and in Normal Control Subjects," *American Journal of Psychiatry,* 145: 1133–1137.

Starr, P., "Atherosclerosis, Hypothyroidism, and Thyroid Hormone Therapy," *Advances in Lipid Research,* 16: 345–371.

Stavig, G. R.; Leonard, A. R.; Igra, A.; & Felten, P., "Indices of Relative Body Weight and Ideal Weight Charts," *Journal of Chronic Disease,* 37(4): 255–262.

Stoffer, S. S., "Menstrual Disorders and Mild Thyroid Insufficiency: Intriguing Cases Suggesting an Association," *Postgraduate Medicine,* 72(2): 75–81.

Surks, M. I., & Ocampo, E., "Subclinical Thyroid Disease," *The American Journal of Medicine,* 100: 217–223.

Taaffe, D. R.; Thompson, J.; Butterfield, G.; & Marcus, R., "Accuracy of Equations to Predict Basal Metabolic Rate in Older Women," *Journal of the American Dietetic Association,* 95(12): 1387–1392.

Takeda, T.; Suzuki, S.; Liu, R.; & DeGroot, L. J., "Triiodothyroacetic Acid Has Unique Potential for Therapy of Resistance to Thyroid Hormone," *Journal of Clinical Endocrinology and Metabolism,* 80: 2033–2040.

Tokunaga, K.; Matsuzawa, Y.; Kotani, K.; Keno, Y.; Kobatake, T.; Fujioka, S.; & Tarui, S., "Ideal Body Weight Estimated from the Body Mass Index with the Lowest Morbidity," *International Journal of Obesity,* 15: 1–5.

Valenta, L. J., & Elias, A. N., "How to Detect Hypothyroidism When Screening Tests Are Normal," *Postgraduate Medicine,* 74(2): 267–274.

Van Lanschot, J. J. B.; Feenstra, B. W. A.; Vermeij, C. G.; & Bruining, H. A., "Calculation versus Measurement of Total Energy Expenditure," *Critical Care Medicine,* 14(11): 981–985.

Walsh, B. J., & Morley, T. F., "Comparison of Three Methods of Determining Oxygen Consumption and Resting Energy Expenditure," *Journal of the American Osteopathic Association,* 89(1): 43–46.

Weigley, E. S., "Average? Ideal? Desirable? A Brief Overview of Height-Weight Tables in the United States," *Journal of the American Dietetic Association,* 84(4): 417–423.

Westphal, S. A., "Unusual Presentations of Hypothyroidism," *The American Journal of Medical Sciences,* 314(5): 333–337.

Whybrow, P. C.; Prange, A. J., Jr.; Treadway, C. R.; & Hill, C., "Mental Changes Accompanying Thyroid Gland Dysfunction," *Archives of General Psychiatry,* 20: 48–63.

Wiberg, G. S.; Devlin, W. F.; Stephenson, N. R.; Carter, J. R.; & Bayne, A. J., "A Comparison of the Thyroxine: Tri-iodothyronine Content and Biological Activity of Thyroid from Various Species," *Journal of Pharmacy and Pharmacology,* 14: 777–783.

Williams, A. D.; Meister, L.; & Florsheim, W. H., "Chemical Identification of Defective Thyroid Preparations," *Journal of Pharmaceutical Sciences,* 52(9): 833–839.

Woeber, K. A., "Subclinical Thyroid Dysfunction," *Archives of Internal Medicine,* 157: 1065–1068.

Wolfstein, R. S., "Dietary Cholesterol and Atherosclerosis," *The Western Journal of Medicine,* 146(5): 621–622.

Wren, J. C., "Thyroid Function and Coronary Atherosclerosis," *Journal of the American Geriatrics Society,* 16(6): 696–704.

Zulewski, H.; Muller, B.; Exer, P.; Miserez, A. R.; & Staub, J., "Estimation of Tissue Hypothyroidism by a New Clinical Score: Evaluation of Patients with Various Grades of Hypothyroidism and Controls," *Journal of Clinical Endocrinology and Metabolism,* 82(3): 771–776.

Appendix G: Recommended Calorie Books

If your tastes run beyond the selection of foods in Chapter 12 there are several calorie books I recommend.

Duyff, Robert Larson, *Complete Food and Nutrition Guide.* Chronimed Publishing, 1998.

Natow, Annette B., and Heslin, Jo-Ann, *The Most Complete Food Counter.* Pocket Books, 1999.

Netzer, Corrine T., *The Dieter's Calorie Counter.* Dell Trade Paperback, 1998.

Thompson Pennington, Jean A., *The Essential Guide to Nutrition and the Foods We Eat.* HarperCollins, 1999.

Appendix H: Other Reading

These are books that deal with the same general subject matter. They will give you further information, although I don't necessarily agree with their total content.

Arem, Ridha, *The Thyroid Solution.* Ballantine Books, 1999.

Barnes, Broda O., and Galton, Lawrence, *Hypothyroidism: The Unsuspected Illness.* Thomas Y. Crowell Co., 1976.

Rosenthal, M. Sara, *The Thyroid Sourcebook.* Lowell House, 1998.

Rubenfeld, Sheldon, *Could It Be My Thyroid?* The Thyroid Society for Education and Research, 1996.

Appendix I: Sample Daily Menus

These are not specific recommendations but rather examples of what a typical 1,000-calorie daily diet might look like. I obviously chose what would please me (and it has) when dieting.

EXAMPLE ONE

Breakfast

One Serving (1 cup) Kellogg's Raisin Bran	200 calories
4 oz. Milk 2% fat	64 calories
1 cup Coffee with 1 oz. Milk 2% fat	16 calories

Lunch

Stouffer's Lean Cuisine Chicken in Peanut Sauce	290 calories
Diet Soda	0 calories

Dinner

8 oz. Orange Roughy, broiled with spices	176 calories

½ cup Le Sueur Early Peas (canned)	60 calories
½ cup SW Small Whole Carrots (canned)	30 calories
Salad	
4 Large Leaves of Romaine Lettuce	12 calories
4 Tablespoons Weight Watchers Caesar	
Salad Dressing	20 calories
1 cup Jell-O, Sugar Free	20 calories
1 cup Coffee with 1 oz. Milk 2% fat	16 calories

Total for the Day **904 calories**

Notes on Example One

1. The breakfast is cereal I strongly recommend (see Chapter 12). A variety of cereals will fill the bill.
2. Lunch is a frozen meal, which should prove quite adequate.
3. Dinner is actually a large serving of fish with sufficient vegetables and a salad. The fish serving size is probably bigger than the portion served in many restaurants. You can broil the fish or make it in a skillet with one of the nonstick sprays. You can jazz it up with spices, garlic, or a little Worcestershire sauce, and you don't have to count their calories.
4. The canned veggies make it easy to count their calories.
5. The salad is a real find. The quantity is large, the calories are only 32, and it happens to be quite tasty. If you prefer another kind of lettuce, use it.
6. You even get a dessert. It's not strawberry cheesecake, but it's not bad either.
7. I have intentionally chosen some items that are not in the food lists in Chapter 12 to show that leeway is certainly permitted.
8. The total for the day is 96 calories less than 1,000, so you can make up those calories with a snack or add that many to another day. Don't forget to put 96 on your Excess Calo-

rie Sheet with a minus sign in front. I purposely went under 1,000 to demonstrate that you can have a substantial menu and still be below 1,000 calories.

EXAMPLE TWO

Breakfast

6 oz. Tomato Juice	35 calories
½ cup Kellogg's All-Bran	50 calories
4 oz. Milk 2% fat	64 calories
½ cup Egg Beaters (Prepared any way)	60 calories
1 cup Coffee with 1 oz. Milk 2% fat	16 calories

Lunch

Healthy Choice Southwestern Grilled Chicken	260 calories
Diet Soda	0 calories

Dinner

6 oz. Tomato Juice	35 calories
Stouffer's Lean Cuisine Hearty Portions	
Salisbury Steak	380 calories
6 oz. Strawberries, frozen	66 calories
1 cup Coffee with 1 oz. Milk 2% fat	16 calories
Total for the Day	**982 calories**

Notes on Example Two

1. We still fell a bit short of 1,000, but there should be plenty to eat.
2. If you mind having tomato juice twice in the day, skip one or try a little Worcestershire sauce in the dinner one.

3. The 1/2 cup of Egg Beaters represents two eggs. One way to prepare them is to scramble them in a skillet using non-stick spray.

4. If you want to add the salad from Example One, you will be over 1,000 by only 14.

EXAMPLE THREE

Breakfast

6 oz. Tomato Juice	35 calories
½ cup Kellogg's All-Bran	50 calories
4 oz. Milk 2% fat	64 calories
½ cup Egg Beaters (Prepared any way)	60 calories
1 cup Coffee with 1 oz. Milk 2% fat	16 calories

Lunch

Salad	
4 Large Leaves of Romaine Lettuce	12 calories
4 Tablespoons Weight Watchers Caesar	
Salad Dressing	20 calories
1 can (6 oz.) Chunk Light Tuna in water	150 calories
Diet Soda	0 calories

Dinner

6 oz. Tomato Juice	35 calories
12 oz. Top Sirloin Steak, Choice	444 calories
1 can Del Monte Mixed Vegetables (16½ ounces)	80 calories
6 oz. Strawberries, frozen	66 calories
1 cup Coffee with 1 oz. Milk 2% fat	16 calories

Total for the Day	**1,048 calories**

Notes on Example Three

1. I've repeated a lot of items from the other examples to demonstrate an easy way to have a varied menu. The lunch and dinner main courses have been changed with a healthy serving of mixed vegetables at dinner added.
2. The substantial 12-ounce steak at dinner, hardly considered a diet course, should surprise as well as please those who crave that type of thing.
3. We've finally gone over 1,000 calories, but only by 48. Be sure to include those on your Excess Calorie Sheet.

Appendix J:
A Patient Fights Back

Although I have repeatedly observed patients whose course of treatment with natural thyroid reinforced my opinion of its superiority over the synthetic variety, perhaps none of their stories were as dramatic as that of another lady, who was *not* a patient of mine. I discovered her "story" while surfing the Internet, and I am grateful that she has allowed me to reprint it here.

Shirley Grose is a freelance writer. Her work involves painstaking research, and her thought processes must be functioning well if she is to do her work properly. In a letter to me she described what had been happening to her.

> Before I knew anything was wrong with me, I tried to leave our small rural town for a business trip. I could not remember how to operate the ATM machine. I was nearly in tears; I then attempted to leave town, to complete my appointment, which was a couple hours' drive. I did not know how to leave town. I could not remember. I thought, of course, I had Alzheimer's disease. Amazingly enough, I hid these things from my family and from my personal physician. Even when my daugh-

ter noticed that I introduced myself to someone whom I
knew quite well, she still did not quite comprehend that
I did not remember this person. I could not remember
friends' and neighbors' names or the names of flowers
and trees.

Her local doctor diagnosed hypothyroidism and prescribed
synthetic thyroid, and the dose was adjusted upward when her
symptoms did not improve. She visited an endocrinologist in a
nearby city, who confirmed her need for large doses of synthetic
thyroid. From day to day Shirley's condition wavered, and she was
dissatisfied with her progress.

Shirley was an avid researcher and knew that natural thyroid
was another drug used for her condition. She was grasping at
straws and was able to convince her local doctor to prescribe it.
There was discernible improvement. A "cyst" had been found in
her neck, and she traveled again to consult another endocrinologist, one with fine credentials.

The second endocrinologist had definite opinions about the
use of natural thyroid and would not prescribe it for her. The letter she wrote to him after her visit is the one I came across on the
Internet by accident. The letter was lengthy, and I have edited
out parts, yet it retains its basic purpose. I have also edited out
the brand name of the synthetic thyroid preparation she took
since it adds nothing to the understanding of the issue.

Dear Doctor ———:

I would like for you to clarify several points which came
up during our recent discussion. You said Armour Natural Thyroid, my thyroid replacement preference, was
impure, not predictably the same strength and old-fash-
ioned. I am concerned about this information because I
have uncovered some research that indicates flaws in this
reasoning.

Would you clarify your statements on Armour Natural Thyroid product? If you feel those statements were valid, can you provide documentation to confirm your opinion that Armour Thyroid is an inferior product to [synthetic thyroid]? Is [synthetic thyroid] really a "new" product or was it "grandfathered in" around 1930? I would like to know why, when I changed to Armour Natural Thyroid, you didn't consider the definite improvement in my health important. I would like to know why you felt I was unqualified to say how my own body felt. Why would you insist upon prescribing a drug that I have tried and does not work well with my body? . . .

Your first statement during my consultation as a new patient was that the Armour Natural Thyroid should be discarded; it was full of impurities, it was of inconsistent strength, and it "went out in the 70s." [Synthetic thyroid] was the drug of choice. Armour was clearly inferior. I explained that I felt better on the Armour Thyroid. You ordered me to throw the Armour Natural Thyroid away and take the [synthetic thyroid] dosage you prescribed. You said that a TSH test would not be valid if taken while on Armour Natural Thyroid. Can you document this last statement? I understand the TSH is considered one objective measurement for thyroid supplementation; however, I question the inference that a patient's subjective opinion is unimportant. You seem to disregard how your patients feel. Have there been any major published studies indicating which product the health consumer preferred? Customers have apparently had no choice in thyroid medication in most instances. Therefore, sales volume is not indicative of customer preference. Also, does the [synthetic thyroid] company fund or in any way contribute to organizations to which you belong or to the university itself? If so, does this influence your decision to singularly prescribe [synthetic thyroid]?

At the end of my appointment, when you began to write my prescription for [synthetic thyroid], I indicated that would not be necessary. You asked, "Why?" I said I was continuing with the Armour Thyroid at the dosage my family physician had prescribed. Your response was, "You don't need to return, do you?" I said, "No, I don't." You further explained you did not use the Armour Natural Thyroid, and you would not treat me if I continued taking it.

Do you refuse to treat thyroid cancer patients who refuse to take [synthetic thyroid]? Should I develop thyroid cancer at some point in the future, would you refuse treatment to me on the basis that I chose not to take [synthetic thyroid]? Can you legally refuse to treat a patient who has thyroid cancer because the patient takes Armour Natural Thyroid? Why should I or any patient be intimidated into taking what they feel is an inferior product? Why should I or any patient suffer a lesser quality of life because of physician bias for a particular brand name? . . .

I would sincerely appreciate an answer with documentation in writing about the statements you have made about [synthetic thyroid] and Armour Thyroid. I feel these are important questions, not only for me, but for the future physicians ———— University educates. These future doctors, including the student who took my thyroid history, have not been given complete information, which would allow them and their patients to make educated decisions about their health and their lives.

Sincerely,
Shirley E. Grose

In her letter to me, Shirley went on to describe the contrast in her life before and after taking the proper dosage of natural thyroid hormone:

When the medicine finally took effect, I felt like I was standing in the middle of a tornado's aftermath. I could see nothing standing around me. My life had been destroyed. My driving license had run out six months previously, my garbage was piled up for lack of payment, my fire insurance had been canceled for nonpayment. . . . I had to relearn basic math skills that revolved around my job. I aged overnight. I reached for my hair and it fell out in my hands. I had been athletic with a good body. Within three months my body swelled to the point where I wore only large, loose dresses. At one point, I could not walk the short distance to my car. I walked to the bathroom, sometimes ate something when I could force it down, and I slept deeply for all but about one hour a day in the first two months after diagnosis. I could not bear the sound of the phone, nor could I withstand the slightest stress. The depression was frighteningly deep. . . .

[My current doctor] gradually increased the natural thyroid. The recovery was not instant, but occurred over a year-and-one-half span, but one day on Armour natural thyroid was more potent than the two months on [synthetic thyroid]. My heart "buzzed" with [synthetic thyroid], for lack of a better word; it calmed and worked smoothly with Armour natural thyroid. My weight fell off slowly. . . .

The last time that I spoke to her, Shirley told me she was feeling just fine.

Index

ALSO AVAILABLE FROM WARNER BOOKS

DOCTOR, WHAT SHOULD I EAT?
Nutrition Prescriptions for Ailments in Which Diet Can Really Make a Difference
by Isadore Rosenfeld, M.D.

Isadore Rosenfeld cuts through nutritional hype, myths, and trends to offer specific food recommendations to treat more than fifty common health conditions, including Parkinson's disease, infertility, heart disease, pms, jet lag, and multiple sclerosis. Based on the latest research and supplemented with sensible menus and nutrition charts, this *New York Times* bestseller offers sound, accessible advice to help maintain good health.

"Extraordinary. . . I'm giving it five stars."
—Ann Landers

30 LOW-FAT VEGETARIAN MEALS IN 30 MINUTES
by Faye Levy

You can cook it tasty…cook it fast…and cook it *100% vegetarian*. It's easy with Faye Levy's 100 low-fat, low-cost, fast-fixing, and boldly seasoned vegetarian dishes. Here are recipes that focus on pasta, beans, rice and other grains, one-pot menus, soups, salads, and fruit desserts—all bursting with flavor. Faye will guide you step by quick step through irresistibly delicious and healthy menus that will save you time and money!

KATHY SMITH'S WALKFIT™ FOR A BETTER BODY
Convenient Flexible Inexpensive Effective Fun
by Kathy Smith with Susanna Levin

The star of America's bestselling fitness videos, Kathy Smith presents WALKFIT™, a complete program based on the safest and most natural exercise of all. It is for people who don't have time to exercise, can't always get to the gym, or don't want to be bothered with expensive equipment. From warm-up stretches to sure-fire techniques for building speed, there is specific advice for seniors, teens, fitness buffs, the overweight, and everyone in between—including expectant and new moms.